The Neck Pain Guide

Answering Your Most Common Questions About Neck Pain, Diagnosis, and Treatment

GEORGE M. GHOBRIAL, M.D.

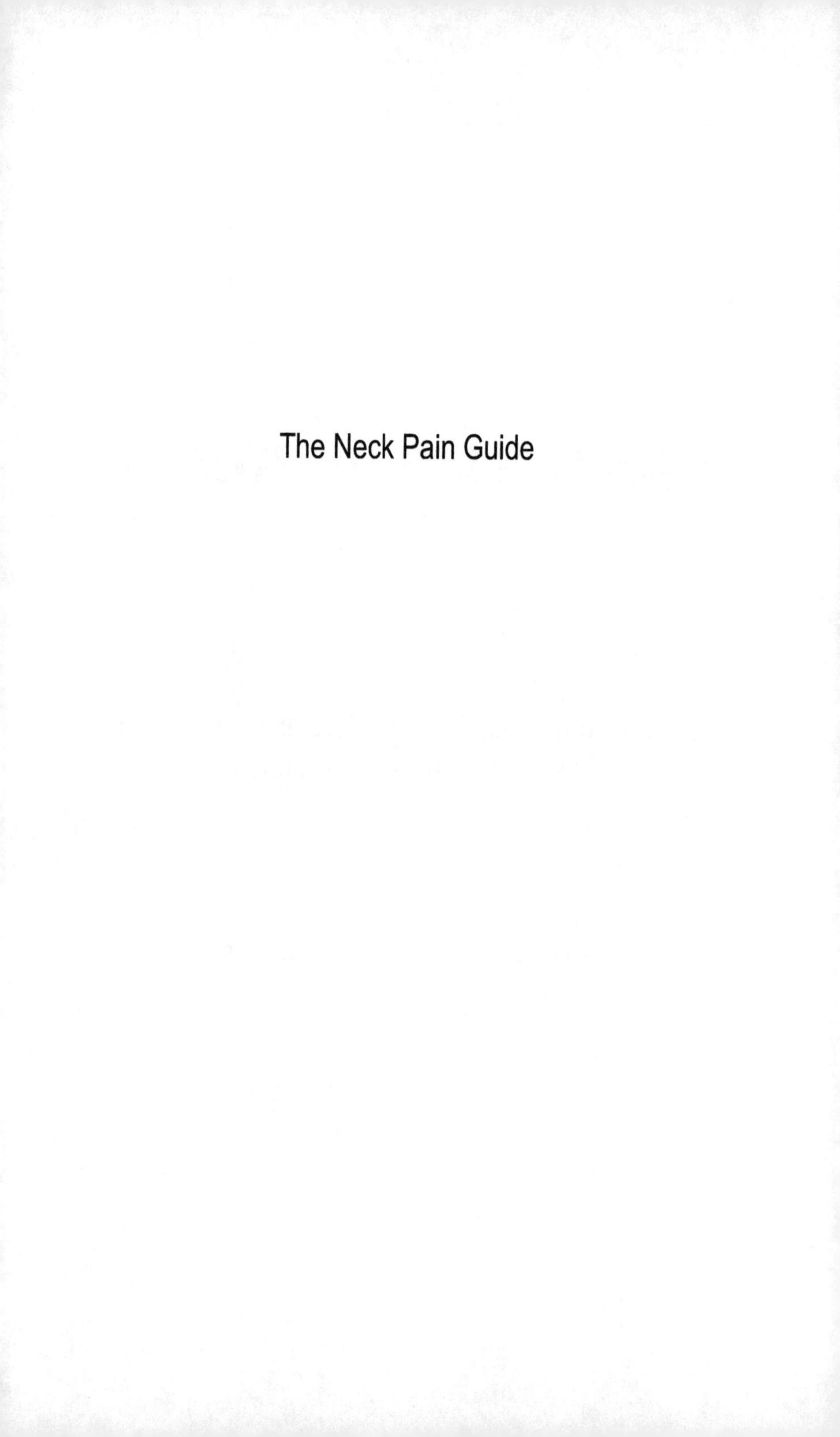

The Neck Pain Guide

Copyright © 2020 by George M. Ghobrial, M.D.

All rights reserved. No part of this book may be reproduced in any form or by any electronic or mechanical means, including information storage and retrieval systems, without permission in writing from the publisher, except by reviewers, who may quote brief passages in a review. This book may not be reproduced, copied, transmitted, or stored in part or in whole, without the written consent of the author. The information in this book is not meant to represent or serve as a substitute for medical care. The data contained herein is meant for educational and entertainment purposes only. This book does not serve as a warranty or guarantee of the completeness or accuracy of this information. The content presented in this book is not a substitute for medical care by a physician or trained healthcare professional, and should not be used for self-diagnosis, primary medical advice, or medical treatment.

ISBN (Paperback Edition) - 9781949148039
Library of Congress Control Number 2020902579

Ilustrated and Edited by George M. Ghobrial, M.D.

Printed and Bound in USA
First Edition First Printing

Published by Weatherly Press LLC
P.O. Box 1071
Pikeville, KY, USA 41502

10 9 8 7 6 5 4 3 2 1

For Michelle,

Alexander, Nicholas, and Timothy

Preface

Neck pain is a common problem, and a major cause of disability in the United States, resulting in almost as many office visits as with low back pain. As such, *The Neck Pain Guide* follows the recently published book, *The Low Back Pain Guide*, with the goal to answer the most common questions about neck pain. In the attempt to provide all new and exciting information about the diagnosis, treatment, and underlying science of neck pain, *The Neck Pain Guide* has expanded to provide a greater emphasis on spinal health in general, in addition to neck pain. In *The Neck Pain Guide,* common symptoms, underlying causes, diagnostic techniques, pain management, surgery, modern experimental treatments and other miscellaneous topics and questions such as the role of 'stem cell' injections are discussed.

This Book Is Ideal For Educating All Audiences With Spinal Pain, With An Emphasis On Neck Pain

This book is ideal for all audiences interested in learning more about the basics of neck pain management, modern healthcare treatments, and a strategy to alleviate pain. Having a medical background is not necessary to understand this book as the goal of this work is to educate patients and provide them with all the information in the same place, and to organize that information into a question-and-answer reference. Since not everyone has the precious free time to read lengthy nonfiction books on a single technical subject, this book is organized to allow for questions and topics to be more rapidly found among the table of contents and index, directing the reader to a helpful explanation and illustration.

Despite being a highly prevalent healthcare problem in North America (also worldwide), there are no comprehensive, patient-centered books that cover the full scope of modern back pain management, which was the motivation for providing *The Low Back Pain Guide,* and later, *The Neck Pain Guide.* Also, unlike the majority of patient-centered educational materials, a truly unique perspective is shared, which is that of a neurosurgeon with expertise and fellowship training in spinal surgery. This book will emphasize non-surgical treatments, since they comprise the majority of spinal care.

A Handbook of Available Neck and Back Pain Treatments

A wealth of information on neck pain is available. With any educational information, (books, articles online, etc...) conscious and unconscious bias due to the authors area of expertise and perspective can redirect the reader towards a particular treatment or product, or similarly steer them away from other treatments. The astute reader must then proceed cautiously whenever advertising is combined with promises; where anyone looks, there are cures. In any case, carefully consider all of the options and alternatives. Use this book to help you explore and understand as many alternatives as possible.

Healthcare Is A Marketplace: Carefully Examine The Merits And Claims Of Each And Every Treatment

The unique healthcare environment that we live in can make it difficult for patients to confidently make independent heathcare decisions. That is partly due to the overwhelming selection of novel treatment options available for neck pain. These products are all vying to meet the demands of our growing and aging US population. Moreover, the market is rife with products that make bold claims, surpassing even the greatest of patient expectations. Marketing a product as curative or as a means to become *pain free*, are prime examples. Indeed, it is quite a daunting marketplace when all participants line up in response to claims of the best treatments. And so, it is often terrifying to make that decision alone. Therefore, it is important to identify someone as early as possible that can help you navigate this process. This advice can be beneficial with navigating any healthcare problem, and it works even better when this person is identified in advance. This is helpful because in matters of severe pain, it is not always possible to remain objective and make the best decisions.

Understand The Fundamental Questions To Ask

Often issues can arise for patients that are vague enough that the starting point in the process of seaking treatment is not even known. Where would the problem-solver begin? Also, other issues come into play such as who to consult for assistance, what is a reasonable price, and what is the typical durability of the product or service being sold (in other words, how long does that service or product last before this issue may arise again)?[1] What are the essential questions one should ask before any service? In one regard, neck pain is simpler in that the question of 'replace or repair' is least often ever a consideration. In fact, as you will read later on, the option to surgically replace a disc in the spine is a rare treatment option and reserved primarily for patients with arm pain symptoms that have met a specific set of criteria through a spinal surgery evaluation- in other terms, a small percentage of patients.[2]

An Ocean of Potential Causes of Neck And Back Pain

Moving forward to the process of process of getting treatment ultimately leads to the fundamental problem and major hurdle to self-diagnosis of neck pain. There are many causes of neck pain, and many more causes of neck and back pain, and very few ways to definitively identify the source. To the author, the diagnostic process is one of the fascinating aspects of modern spinal medicine.

---

1 *In medicine, the term 'durability' describes how long a treatment effect will last.*

2 *A fraction of patients with predominantly arm pain symptoms and other specific criteria met on imaging, may be a candidate for cervical disc replacement, a treatment for cervical radiculopathy (painful cervical nerve compression), which is discussed in the section on surgery.*

The definitive diagnosis of the ailment causing the underlying back or neck pain issue may not come due to the presence of multiple pain generators. This means that multiple problems are often simultaneously generating pain across multiple levels or anatomical locations within and adjacent to the spine, assuming the pain is arising from the spine to begin with. In this book, the numerous causes of neck pain due to spinal and non-spinal pain generators will be discussed, as well as options for diagnosis. This will include practical assistance with understanding the rationale for using different tools to image the spine and why tests are frequently used to increase diagnostic accuracy, and also when they are less likely to be helpful.

Challenges To Finding Reliable Sources Of Information On The Internet

Another major challenge is in navigating the emerging platforms for new educational material. Social media and targeted advertising has grown more sophisticated. The healthcare market is like any other giant market- even browsing habits and advertising content are often tailored to grab your attention, or to direct you to a particular product or treatment.

Confidently evaluating a treatment for a disease process requires an understanding of evidence-based medicine and the terminology. In the context of medicine, understanding terms such as efficacy, quality, reliability, accuracy, significance, correlation, and the strength of a recommendation, are invaluable as a sound understanding of these issues allows us to ask the most helpful questions. This goes a long way because this will remind the reader that not all treatments are the same (in terms of quality as well), and indications for the use of a particular treatment can be narrow.

Some patients may then begin to ask certain questions such as , "How do I know this treatment will work?" Or, "What is the likelihood that this treatment will work?", and "How long will this treatment work?" The last question is seldomly asked, but arguably the most pertinent question, because most spinal pain attributed to degenerative conditions is an ongoing life process, meaning that it is more often lessened than cured. The reader will be even more surprised that evidence of promising results from the latest research study on the news may be irrelevant for many patients. Nonetheless, these questions and others lead to the issue of how to assess medical studies, which for brevity can only be very concisely discussed in this book. This is a very complex subject, but even understanding a few of the most basic research principles of translational medicine[3] will help any patient gain a far greater insight into healthcare than most patients.

How Can I Assess The 'Quality' Of Medical Treatments And Evidence?

Again, the issues with deciding which treatment has the best 'record' is understanding that not all statements about a medical product are backed by medical studies of the same quality (grade). If you are unfamiliar with grading medical evidence, it all comes from study design, and the multimillion dollar expense of the most well-designed studies. Basically, the better the information, the better the study design which cannot be performed to answer every medical question, frankly because it is impossible to do so. The best study designs such as the double-blinded, placebo-controlled, randomized, clinical trials typically are the most expensive, require the greatest number of personel, greatest time commitment, and extensive use of independent regulator oversight to ethically com-

3 *Translational medicine refers to the ethical incorporation of laboratory and clinical research. Or, it is the concept of bringing knowledge from the 'bench to the bedside' (a phrase coined by Spencer King, M.D., online https://www.ahajournals.org/doi/full/10.1161/ 01.cir.93.9.1621 May 1, 1996).*

plete. These are the studies that generally can provide via interpretation of the results, the best recommendations for treatment, where available. And since these studies are few and far between, how do we assess the other studies? Even so, how well were the studies designed?

Professional Healthcare Assistence Will Be Eventually Required

It becomes clear that unless you have a background in the medical field, chances are you will need professional guidance at some point for your neck pain. This book can bring you as closed to informed as possible. In many instances, this book can help you draw the line between self-education and professional consultation.

Question and Answer Format For Learning About Spinal Diseases And Treatment Options

This book is organized as a reference material into the common and uncommon questions asked by patients about neck pain. It is organized chronologically into five sections. The first section is an introduction on the topic of neck pain, followed by a guide to early neck pain management, spinal imaging and tests, and available treatment options which can include surgery or early medical treatments (nonsurgical). Specialized topics are found in the final section, which provide a guide to assess healthcare treatments. For example, at the onset of developing neck discomfort, while staring at a cell phone all day, or while sitting on a plane, uncomfortably reading a book in your lap, has the reader ever wondered what might be the causes and consequences? A review of the concerns and research on this subject, ergonomics, and 'text-neck' are briefly included.

In the appendix, various useful tools and guides for a number of miscellaneous topics are included. Also, a helpful reference sheet has been created for patients to outline your back and neck history. Keeping this journal or some kind of record is important. Patients accumulate far too many treatments- getting lost in the history of medications, office visits, injections, and various other therapies and diagnostic tests over time.

Again, this book was designed for anyone to be able to pick up and use. If you made it this far, keep reading, as you are already be well on your way to understanding modern neck pain management and hopefully this will get you on the road to pain relief!

Introduction

Neck pain, also called *cervicalgia*, is defined as regional pain occuring between the base of the skull, upper torso (thoracic spine)[4], and extending outwards to the margin of the shoulders (Fig. I). This is one of the most common medical problems facing everyone in their lives, regardless of health, fitness level, occupation, or status in society. At any given time, more than 15% of people report that they have low back and neck pain. In fact, this is so common that it is referred to as part of *the human experience*. Of course, this is just another way of saying that this is part of life, or part of growing older. However, this should not be interpreted as a a lack of concern for your well-being.

---

4 *Adapted From American Academy of Orthopedic Surgeons, https://orthoinfo.aaos.org/en/diseases--conditions/neck-pain*

THE BOUNDARIES OF NECK PAIN EXTEND BEYOND THE NECK

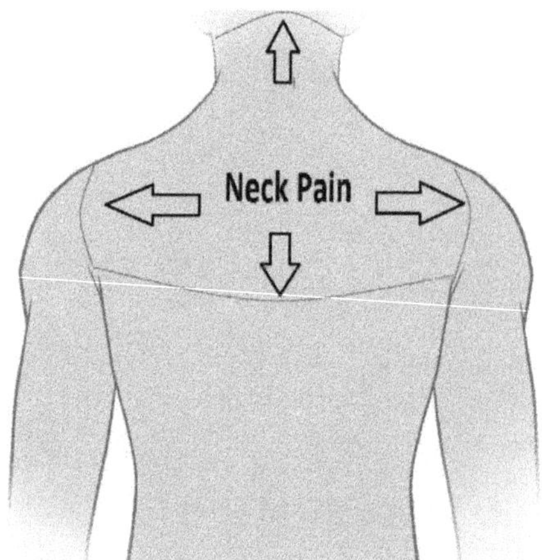

Figure I. Neck pain can extend beyond the neck to the base of the skull, the mid thoracic spine, and just to the margins of the shoulders. Basically, muscle spasms are the most common cause of neck pain, and many neck muscles extend to the upper spine, base of the skull, and outer limits of the clavicle.

Why is Neck Pain So Common?

There are numerous causes of neck pain. Yet, the single most common reason for the increased prevalence of neck pain is that the population is aging. The degeneration of our collective joints occurs at a steady rate. So, if people are living longer, more joints reach a critical point where disabling pain occurs. Osteoarthropathy is a general term that refers to any disease of the joints, it is similar to the term arthritis, and spondylosis is a general term for arthritic or degenerative conditions of the spine. Degenerative osteoarthropathy encompasses the majority of cases, which is a broad category of joint conditions afflicting older patients. Other reasons for increases in neck pain are a result of observation and technology. Major changes in our healthcare system in the past twenty years have led to an increased use of electronic medical records, which, in tandem with an incredible US population growth and increases in access to healthcare- all lead to the increased number of patients identified with new onset neck pain in the United States. To summarize, when we look more frequently and more thoroughly for a disease, we tend to find more of that disease.

Analogies

Analogies help summarize some incredibly complex processes, and they can often bring you much closer to understanding what is going on with your medical problems and treatment, and for some, providing more clarity than if the physician spent an hour describing everything in detail. However, analogies have major limitations. The biggest one is informed consent, which requires the understanding of specific concepts such as certain specific risks. Returning to analogies, consider the following:

"The spine is like the frame of a car, that helps you get from point A to point B. The vertebrae are the main weight-bearing bones of the spine, and are separated by discs that provide cushioning and flexibility. The discs also distribute shock and protect the nerves and spinal cord within. A car, like the human body, has its frame also, and getting from point A to point B subjects many parts to wear- tires, brakes, struts, shocks, and more. However, in the spine, 'factory(OEM)', or original parts, you will keep those factory original parts (in the spine) for all 80 or so years of your life. Tires can be swapped out in the shop, so can oil, filters, and every other part for that matter, but in general, there is no way to replace parts of the spine.[5] The discs are permanent, and they will wear out - slowly becoming stiffer, then thinner, allowing the segments of bone in your spine to get closer and closer to each other, until eventually there will be 'bone-on-bone' contact. In keeping with the same analogy, this is like driving on rims without any tires."

The analogy above does not bring the patient any closer to understanding the concepts of disc degeneration and spondylosis, Also, it does not raise understanding of the available surgical and non-surgical treatment options, and the risks of these treatments. Yet, by and large, analogies help plenty of patients get a better handle on what is going on. Not every patient can be taught all of what was learned in residency in a few office visits.

Other Common Analogies of The Spine

- Brick and Mortar: The vertebrae are the bricks and the mortar are the discs. This is a basic analogy of the arrangement of the spinal column.

- Jelly Donuts: A common reference to a disc herniation (which will be reviewed in detail in the appropriate chapters). A disc has a tough, round exterior, called the *annulus fibrosus*, and the internal gelatinous contents are called the *nucleus pulposus*, which is like a the jelly in a donut. When the disc herniates, the gelatinous contents may enter the spinal canal and

---

5 *Truthfully, this analogy worked well until the cervical disc replacement procedure became possible. However, most people are not candidates for this procedure and this will be discussed in detail later. For the most part, the analogy above still holds true that there are no replacements to the parts of the spine.*

irritate the nerve, thus exiting the donut.

- Tire: This is another common reference to describe a disc herniation. The disc provides cushioning, similar to a tire on a car. Needless to say, lose air in the tire, bad things are in store for the rest of the car. Air cannot be pumped into the disc.

Technology and New Treatment Options

As we have mentioned, neck pain is becoming more common, and people are living longer, which means that more patients are getting treatment for their neck pain. Another reason for the growth in neck pain treatment is the development of new treatment therapies and increased safety of existing treatments, which have the effect of increasing general access of the public to these treatments. From a technology standpoint, it is far easier to treat pain than to cure it. Even so, it is hard to effectively control pain in many instances. Unfortunately, it is unlikely that any time soon there will be a cure for neck pain, just as there is not a cure for LBP, or a way to stop degenerative joint diseases.

The most common spinal and non-spinal causes of neck pain from the very frequent to the rare causes will be discussed in the chapters below. As you will read in this book, the bones, discs, joints, and ligaments of the spine are not always the source of the neck pain.

One of the most common causes of chronic neck pain is chronic muscular strain, which is a stiff, painful neck- a pulled muscle. An MRI cannot diagnose routine muscle strain. Often patients seek help for chronic muscle strain, and eventually make their way to pain management specialists and spinal surgeons for treatment. This common practice actually highlights two key points, and is not in any way a criticism. The first point is that there isn't a very good diagnostic test and treatment pathway for the most common cause of neck pain, which is muscle strain. The second point is that with increased technology, we can identify more drivers of neck pain, and more treatments for these causes of neck pain. So, if the problem cannot be diagnosed, or alleviated, or too many diagnoses are identified, then patients are going to spend more time in our healthcare system seeking various specialists and treatments, with persistent neck pain. Healthcare is rapidly becoming more complex and confusing to someone without a medical background, and for neck pain care, this is partly due to the aforementioned number of treatments and causes of neck pain.

If this book is able to help you, it will explain some of the common misconceptions about neck pain that exist. It is not a do-it-yourself manual, neither is it primarily a self-help manual. Rather, this book should be used as a helpful reference, in tandem with the advice and consultation from your trusted physician or other healthcare provider.

Healthcare today requires numerous appointments, interspersed with lengthy waiting periods. While that is disheartening to be in pain and not get a speedy resolution, the unintended benefit is that most patients with neck pain due to a disc herniation or episode of muscular strain will experience the resolution or partial improvement of that painful episode within the first three months. Have you ever wondered why so many treatments require a 3 month wait period or greater, prior to getting approval by insurance? Waiting often allows you to experience pain resolution before obtaining a more aggressive treatment.

When would it be an appropriate time to accelerate a workup for neck pain? When is it appropriate to obtain imaging, if many people needlessly obtain imaging in the early period? Imaging reports are more commonly available to patients for review, and certainly create confusion due to the long and cryptic description used by radiologists to describe the spinal imaging study.[6] Most patients arrive in the neurosurgical clinic with just a basic understanding that neck pain always arises from the spine itself.

Advanced Imaging: Double-Edged Sword

At the moment, the most advanced diagnostic imaging study of the neck is an MRI, which stands for magnetic resonance imaging, and it can provide a highly detailed picture of the spine. Recall that the MRI does not provide diagnostic detail to highlight an active cause of muscle strain, except in the most severe circumstances. Rarely, some academic centers provide MRI studies that can emphasize muscle strain to some degree of accuracy, which is after all the most common cause of neck pain. Again, recall that the radiologists provide a complex report intended for specialists familiar with the terms and their implications as they apply to their patients, and not intended for the general audiences to understand.

Degenerative Diseases Are A Lifelong Process

When a patient receives their first MRI report, chances are, that this report contains a description of a degenerative 'disease'. However, as eluded to in the above section about advanced imaging, 'degeneration' in most cases is no more than a description of the aging spine.

---

6 A scientific description of your imaging report are collectively called *findings*. The radiologist summarizes this lengthy description in what is known as an *impression*.

Is This Spinal Problem Due to An Accident?

The chief problem with answering this question is that stenosis, disc herniations, and other problems that are considered 'degenerative spinal pathologies' are found with a high frequency in patients without back or neck pain. A convincing argument can be successfully made that degeneration of the spine is just a natural process of aging of the intervertebral disc, and usually not the chief cause of the new onset of back and neck pain. **Therefore, the diagnosis of degenerative disc disease and herniated discs in the process of working up back and neck pain does not establish a cause and effect relationship**. Many patients ask if a spinal degenerative condition identified on MRI resulted from an injury. Hypothetically, if two-thirds of the general population already have a condition, then this is a very tenuous conclusion to make from looking at one MRI. If any conclusions are to be made, many other factors must be taken into consideration.

Conclusions

Degenerative disc disease is a catch-all phrase encompassing the naturally-occuring process of spinal aging, just like spondylosis.[7] It is often a driver of pain, but this is often difficult to prove. A spine surgeon, or other spine specialist listens to you, and after a careful examination, decides a care plan, which may or may not include imaging, along with other non-surgical treatment measures. Most neck or low back pain is due to muscle strain, and improves without surgery. Since there is no form of diagnostic imaging for muscle strain, it is common to want to reject muscle strain in favor

---

7 *Many definitions of spondylosis include the descriptive phrase, 'wear-and-tear'.*

of diseases that can be clearly defined and evaluated with imaging, i.e. with an MRI showing a lumbar disc bulge. Ultimately, your response to treatment of a neck pain flare-up and the natural course of improvement over time will usually serve as confirmation of a muscle strain. Most flare-ups of neck or low back pain will improve without treatment.

Therefore, obtaining an imaging study prematurely may unlock the path to a long cycle of timely and invasive nonsurgical and surgical treatments. Avoid these if at all possible. A description of these options are found in this book, as the goal of this book is to help demystify as many neck pain treatments as possible.

Regardless, your adventure will be unique, and not all circumstances can be controlled, regardless of how much research you do. Educate yourself about the treatment options for neck pain, including those presented in this book. Consider all of your options and see how this fits your goals and lifestyle. Treatment recommendations for chronic processes that are of relatively low urgency can be tailored to fit your unique lifestyle and values. Your physcian can tailor your treatment in this case to meet your needs and expectations, Discuss these expectations with your care provider before committing to any type of therapy. An increased percentage of your medical education will be web-based. As healthcare has become increasingly more complex, the massive amount of information can be less liberating than hoped. In this book, general strategies for evaluating medical research and online information will be discussed that are applicable to neck pain, low back pain, and strategies to assess treatments in other areas of medicine as well.

George M. Ghobrial, M.D.

Contents

IV: NON-SURGICAL TREATMENT...................221

Section I

Getting Answers

1 What is Neck Pain?

Neck pain requires little introduction, occuring nearly as frequently as low back pain. Neck pain is any discomfort between the base of the skull and upper shoulders and thoracic spine. The distribution of neck pain most often correlates with the insertions and origins of various groups of muscles that support the posture of the cervical spine. Therefore, most of the neck pain that we experience is due to overexertion and is musculoskeletal in nature. Among the cervical, thoracic, and lumbar spine, the cervical spine located in the neck has singularly the greatest range of motion in any particular direction, allowing our head and with it, the freedom to interact with our environment (Fig. 1-1). The reliance of the neck musculature to support the head and cervical spine puts the muscle at risk for injury. Usually, neck pain is the result of 'microtears' in the muscle, that will heal over a short time period with rest. However, repetitive and frequent activities that strain the neck and without sufficient rest, can result in chronic neck pain.

Because the spine is most frequently the focus of an exhaustive and detailed workup for common chronic neck and back pain, the basics will be briefly described below regarding the spine, it's structure and function, and related pain syndromes.

The Cervical Spine In Relation To Your Neck

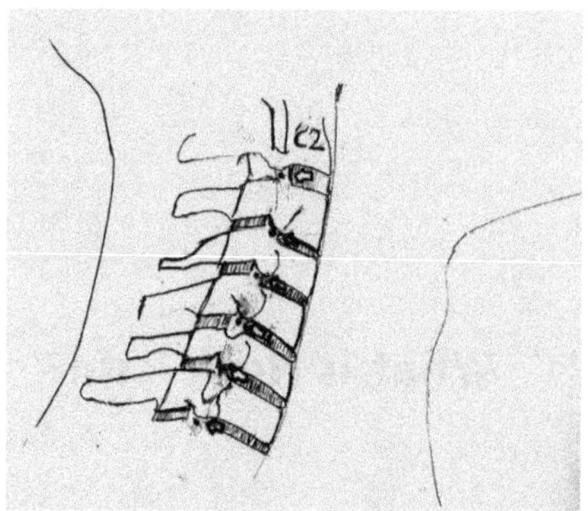

Figure 1-1. The cervical spine consists of seven segments. The second (labelled C2) through seventh cervical vertebra is illustrated above. The cervical nerve roots exit the spine through a bony channel called the neural foramen (small arrows). The margins of the neck are outlined.

The spine provides support and structure to the neck (your 'backbone') and is comprised of blocks of bone called *vertebral bodies*, connected by discs, these are the basic supporting segments of the spine (Fig. 1-2). The cervical spine in the neck is the uppermost region of the spine, comprising 7 segments. These segments form a bony column that articulates with the base of the skull, forming a channel for the spinal cord. The spinal cord is all-important, to say the least. It is carries the voluntary and involuntary (unconscious) electrical impulses that send and receive information between the brain and the body. This includes movement, sensation, balance, pain, as well as bowel, bladder, sexual function, and more.

The Spinal Column

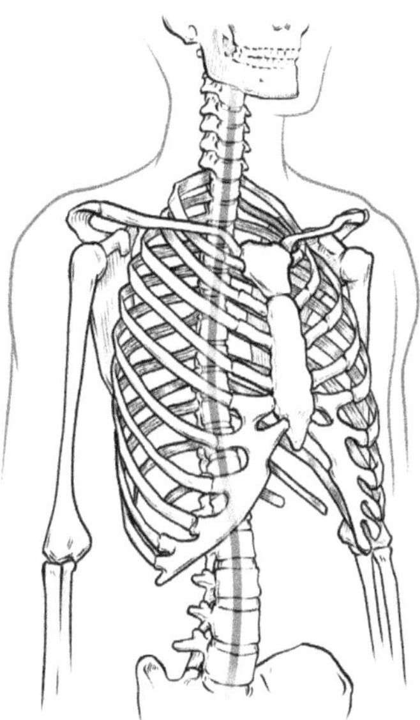

Figure 1-2. The largest component of each spinal segment is a large block of bone called the vertebra.[8] The spinal cord runs throughout the spinal column (broad line). The cervical spinal comprises 7 segments. The thoracic spine is twelve segments, and are unique in that there are twelve associated pairs of ribs that impart additional stability to this region of the spine. The lumbar spine is typically five levels and carries nerves down to the lower extremities. This region is the most common area to be affected by painful problems of disc degeneration due to the increased motion and bearing the weight of the majority of the body. The sacral spine is the lowest part of the spine, and lacks disc segments. Five pairs of sacral nerves travel through the sacrum into the pelvis. The first of those five pairs, S1, forms part of the sciatic nerve.

---

8 *Vertebra is a latin word meaning, 'joint'. When you see the word spelled as vertebrae, it is commonly used as an alternative spelling, but it formally refers to the spelling of the plural form of the word.*

A Pair of Spinal Nerves Exits in Close Proximity to The Vertebral Body and Disc

In between the vertical stack of vertebral bodies are shock absorbing cushions called *intervertebral discs (discs)*. The structure of the spine gives us our upright posture and the discs act as flexible shock absorbers. The discs are made up mostly of water, collagen, and interface with the bone of the vertebral body above and below. In close proximity to the disc is a pair of exiting nerve roots, that sends and receive information to and from the body. These nerves exit through a bony channel called a neural foramen (Fig. 1-3).

Relationship Of The Vertebral Body, and Cervical Disc To Exiting Nerve Roots

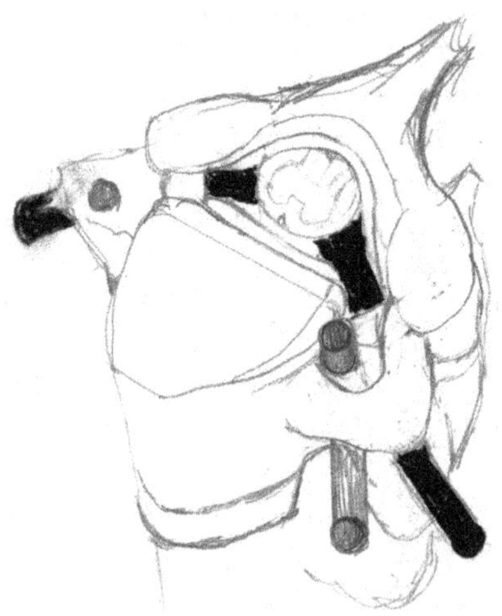

Figure 1-3. The vertebral body is a large block of bone that bears the major-

ity of your weight, and transmits that weight down to your legs. The bone is surrounded by intervertebral discs, which are soft and flexible, functioning as shock absorbers and providing some spinal flexibility. The human spine provides us with an upright posture and is central for walking on two legs. Segments of nerves exit at each level in the neural foramen, which are spaces between joints at each level that serves as entrances and exits for nerve roots (darkened structures). Note the proximity of the cervical disc to the exiting nerve root (arrow).

2 What Are Some of The Underlying Causes of Neck Pain?

There are numerous causes of neck pain. Occasionally, the diagnosis is very difficult to make. However, many important clues can help you narrow down your diagnosis. Generally, neck pain is most often due to inflammation of the muscles and ligaments of the neck, this will improve with rest. Disc disease and disc herniation are types of degenerative conditions of the cervical spine, and are also thought to be a very common cause of neck pain. These are among the most difficult to treat, because to this day, discogenic pain is a controversial diagnosis, lacking an appropriate diagnostic technique to link the disc to the symptoms of cervical disc degeneration which are primarily generalized neck pain.[9] Following that, inflammation of the soft tissues of the neck can cause pain that appears similar to a spinal or muscular problem, and this is called referred pain. Often, adjacent anatomy can cause overlapping symptoms with neck pain, such as degenerative diseases impacting the scapula, shoulder, and clavicle. In the case of a prior traumatic injury, chronic neck pain can be a signs of musculoskeletal strain or sprain, which can heal with rest, or a sign of a problem requiring attention, such as a nonhealing fracture.

Neck Pain Etiologies

Summarized from above, the two most common drivers of neck pain muscles are the ligaments of the neck and the cervical spine itself. In the cervical spine, there are numerous further causes of neck pain that we will briefly list, and describe in greater detail in the following sections.

Cervical Radiculopathy

One important cause of neck pain is related to irritation of the cervical nerves in the neck, called *cervical radiculopathy*. The cervical nerves exit the spine at each level, placing them at risk for painful compression. Compression at the point of nerve exit causes neck pain and pain that can travel down the arm, in a unique pattern. This is typically sharp, and followed by sensory symptoms such as tingling, and is short-lived. Nerve roots that arise from particular regions of the spine, for example, between C4 and C5, which is the C5 nerve, travels to a predictable location in a large percentage of people, supplies (innervates), specific muscles and specific regions of skin near the shoulder. All of these characteris-

---

9 *Peng B, DePalma M. Journal of pain research. 2018: 11 space 2853-2857*

tics such nerve root compression. These will be discussed in detail below as this predictable pattern is studied and hence there are many spinal treatments that effectively address cervical radiculopathy.

Non-Spinal Causes of Neck Pain

Due to the nature of neck pain, there are many causes that are non-spinal. They will be distributed in appropriate locations throughout the book. As you will see in the following list, some of them are concerning medical issues. This is why the author advocates that the reader establishes care with a healthcare specialist who can make sure 'red-flags' are identified. A chapter on red-flag conditions/findings is included in a separate chapter due to the critical nature of identifying these scenarios to limit the delay before one seeks medical advice.

Non-Spinal Causes of Neck Pain

Visceral and Other Sources of Potential Neck Pain:
Thyroid Disease
Infection (eg. sore throat, inflammed lymph glands)
Skin Conditions
Heart Conditions
Regional Degenerative Joint Conditions
Shoulder (rotator cuff, labrum tear, bursitis, etc...)
sternum (chest/'breast bone')
clavicle ('collar bone')

3 What is Disc Degeneration?

An intervertebral disc is located between almost all levels of the mobile spine, with the exception being that between the skull (called the 'occiput') and the first cervical level, as well as the level between the first and second cervical level (C1 and C2). These areas of the cervical spine in the neck are responsible for the majority of the range of motion of the neck. Discs contain a relatively thick outer ring called the annulus, which contains a core, called the nucleus pulposus, which is gelatinous, predominantly water and held together in a matrix of various forms of collagen and connective tissue who binds a larger volume of water. Over time, this soft center dehydrates, losing its water. This is the process of disc degeneration, and is automatic.

Regardless of the person, the spine will slowly age. Again, this happens to everyone. As a result, an adult who has an MRI of their cervical or lumbar spine is going to have to ask themselves what the MRI would look like before their symptoms started. Is it possible that the spine was without any degeneration before the pain began? Unless you are under the age of 20, and most likely, that is not the case, then you are going to find an imaging report describing degenerative diseases. The most common diagnosis patients find on their report is degenerative disc disease (DDD) and spondylosis (Fig. 3-1). It can be difficult for a physician to sometimes convince a patient that a disc that is degenerating is unlikely the cause of the pain, since it is difficult to clearly prove, and also because the problem is classified as a disease.

Genetics is thought to play a role in the rate of disc degeneration and unfortunately, how genetics influences disc degeneration is difficult to determine. It is thought that multiple genes exert varying degrees of influence. Regardless, this part is not something that can be reliably tested for, modified, or proven.

Your lifestyle can have an impact on disc degeneration, just as with any other joint. Obesity can lead to early joint disease, such as knee and hip osteoarthritis. The lumbosacral spine is no different. The cervical spine can be impacted as well. One other modifiable risk factor is thought to be tobacco use, which has been shown to cause numerous health issues, including disc degeneration.

Disc Degeneration Results In Osteophyte Formation And Stenosis

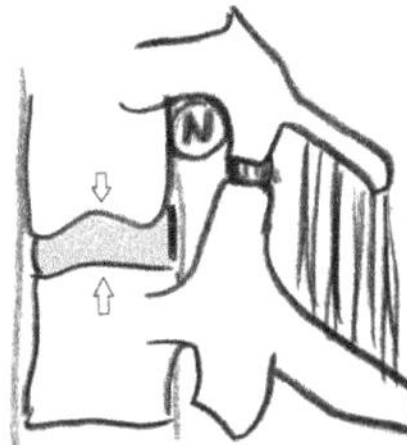

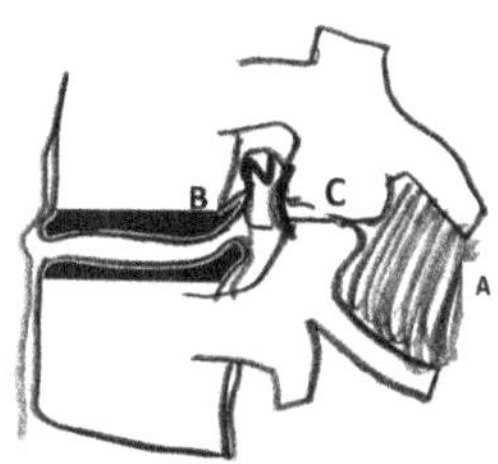

Figure 3-1. Cervical disc degeneration results in shortening of the disc space (left, disc is shaded). Loss of disc height results in increased pressure on the disc space and increased density of the endplate (sclerosis, darkened perimeter of the disc space). This results in endplate changes and osteophyte formation (or spurs, body extensions B), facet hypertrophy(C), ligamentous hypertrophy (A), and ultimately encroachment of the nerve roots (N).

Discogenic Pain

Pain caused by inflammation of the disc is referred to as *discogenic pain.* Discogenic neck pain is a relatively less common source of neck pain when compared to low back pain, and the reason is likely due to the increased biomechanical forces that are transmitted through the lumbosacral spine, which is lower on the *totem pole,* so to speak, carrying the weight of all the vertebrae above. This is in fact why the vertebrae are normally of comparatively increasing size as one travels from the cervical to thoracic and to the lumbar spine. Over time, the older one gets, as discs degenerate, the facet joints, which are paired joints at every spinal level, undergo a similar process of degeneration. These joints can further contribute to neck and back pain. As you can see, degenerative diseases of the spine describe the 'wear-and-tear' that occurs, and the inflammation that causes pain. Given enough time, this process will impact all joints in the body. This is no different than needing to repair parts on your vehicle over time.

Is There a Test That Can Identify a Painful Cervical Disc?

Unfortunately, there still is no consensus regarding a specific test. The same is true for low back pain, thought by many to be caused by the disc (discogenic LBP). Can discography, a study to identify a painful disc be useful? Discography is a procedure where a needle is guided into the center of a particular disc space with the intent to reproduce or increase the pain intensity (Fig. 3-2). Since this procedure itself has been shown to create painful discogenic pain in people without prior discogenic-type pain, it has fallen out of favor with many clinicians due to mixed reviews. How does the disc generate pain? The outer layer of the disc, called the annulus, has pain fibers, which can increase in number with chronic inflammation. Keep in mind that not all abnormal discs are painful!

Cervical Discography

Cervical discography is an x-ray-assisted (fluoroscopic) dye injection of the cervical disc space with the goal for the diagnosis of the painful, problematic (pathologic) degenerated disc (Fig. 3-2). The utility of the cervical discography is a controversial study. In a 2001 review of previously published scientific studies, it fell short of the mark for meeting satisfactory requirements to support use of the procedure for diagnosing neck pain.[10] In some studies, there was up to a 15% increased risk of complication which could include discitis, epidural abscess, epidural hematoma, anterior neck hematoma, spinal cord injury, and quadriplegia. However, some studies found that it was safe and useful, especially when the MRI shows primarily mild degenerative findings in the setting of chronic neck pain.

Cervical Discography

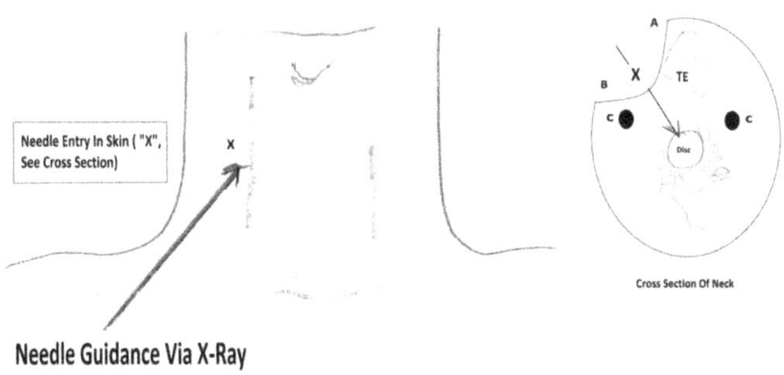

Figure 3-2. Cervical discography : Cervical discography involves the insertion of a needle into the neck (see left illustration above, entry into skin, marked X, into right anterior neck just lateral to trachea). One technical aspect of this procedure involves avoiding the carotid(c) and tracheus and esophagus (TE). The specialist uses x-rays (fluoroscopy) to guide the needle away from the major structures. This is further aided by manually displacing the carotid laterally (B) and trachea medially (A). Suprisingly, the literature is replete with reports of an overall low risk of injury to the critical

10 *Baker RM. Deja vu all over again. The Spine Journal 10 (2010) 736-638.*

structures of the neck. Nonetheless, this procedure is not commonly performed due to the potentially devastating complications and lack of high-quality literature in support of its use. However, this procedure is occasionally performed as some interventionalists attest to the value of this procedure.

4 How Does Disc Degeneration Relate to Spurs and Stenosis?

The discs are approximately 80 percent water. At some point in adolescence, the disc slowly begins the final process of continual dehydration (dessication). Being mostly comprised of water, as the water diffuses out of the disc, the disc loses volume, becoming shorter. To a degree, it is known that constant pressure causes the disc to lose water and become smaller throughout the day, making one shorter. This process reverses while sleeping. However, over its life, the disc is dehydrating and does not retain it's full capacity. This is one of the reasons why someone may believe that they are shorter later in life. In some people, as little as a few millimeters of height loss results in painful nerve compression (Fig. 4-1).

Disc Degeneration And Reactive Changes In The Adjacent Bone

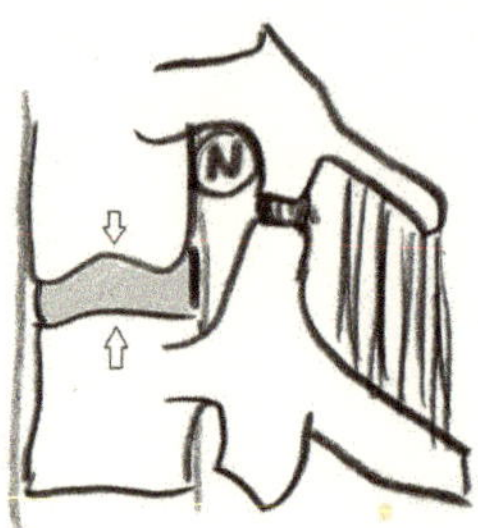

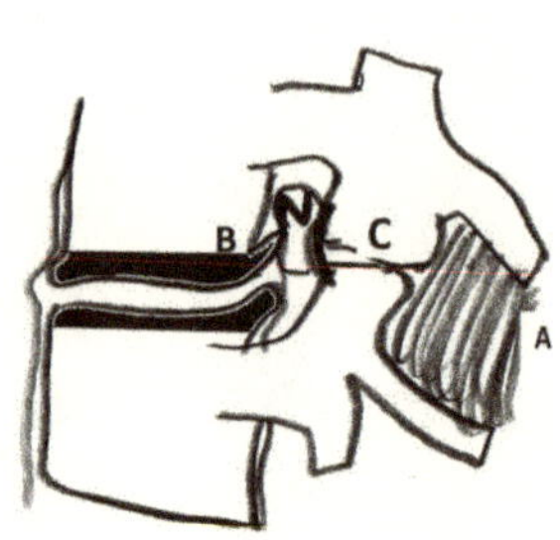

Figure 4-1. The well-hydrated disc space mitigates shock and distributes forces of body weight (normal disc, left figure; a simplified diagram showing a side view of a cross section just off of the midline on either side of the body) providing sufficient space for the exiting nerve (N). Degeneration results in increased pressure within the disc and on the surrounding bone adjacent to the disc space, as well as the formation of new bone (B). The ligaments surrounding the disc lose tension and 'micro-instability' and this spinal level results in changes that increase stability which includes osteophyte formation (B), enlargement of the facets (C), and thickening of the posterior ligaments (A). These processes (A-C) along with the collapse of the disc space can decrease available room for the nerves (N), termed stenosis, and can even result in (nerve compression).

Dehydration may cause cracks to form in the posterior lining of the disc (a radiologist may call it an annular fissure in an MRI report). This lining is called the annulus fibrosus, and separates the disc from the spinal canal, where the nerves course. The annulus is comprised of collagen and is very stiff. It contains less water and degenerates less compared to the disc space. This is important in containing the disc material within the disc space. As the discs degenerate, increased pressure can occur within the disc space, causing herniations of disc material through the annulus (disc herniation) or into the adjacent bone (referred to as a Schmorl's node, which is commonly observed on a lumbar spine MRI report, and less commonly in the cervical spine). Schmorl's nodes can be identified on in both patients with and without symptoms, and once in a while, are characterised on an occasional report as a chronic compression fracture.[11] The discs degenerate, stress occurs on the adjacent bony endplate causing painful inflammation. Inflammation in this region is thought to cause nerve inflammation as well and result in painful signals being sent to the brain, resulting in discogenic pain (Fig 4-2).

Progressive Disc Degeneration Contributes To Osteophyte Formation and Stenosis

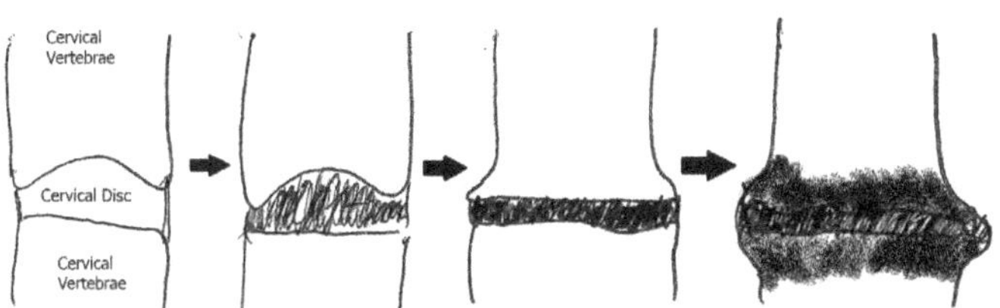

Figure 4-2. Cervical degenerative disc disease (DDD) is present in the majority of adults over the age of 40. The cervical vertebral levels provide structure and functure(left). Disc degeneration is a set of progressive processes marked by a loss of water over time (arrows) in the normal disc

11 *Compression fractures are uncommon in the neck, and in the absence of any recent injury, require further workup. The most common cause is a treatable condition called osteoporosis, which is due to low bone density, and is concerning as one untreated osteoporotic fracture is predictable of several untreated fractures.*

space, which is 80% of the mass of the disc, resulting in encroachment of loss of disc height. Bone spurs form which are areas of new bone growth in attempts to increase spinal stability, along with thickening of the ligaments, and endplate sclerosis. These processes may eventually contribute to neck and arm pain.

Spinal Degeneration Research: 18th Century to Present

The above description of the process of disc degeneration and the many manifestations that occur in the spine have not changed significantly in the past century. Consider one theory of degenerative arthritis by Dr. Julius Wolff, a German surgeon who practiced in the 19th century. He observed that the more weight or forces on a bony surface, the more dense that bone becomes. He theorized that the body reacts to decrease the forces on any one area (the pressure) by enlarging the contact surface. In the process, the bone becomes thicker, and develops bone spurs that increases the surface area of the joint, resulting in decreased pressure over any particular area. The understanding of spondylosis today is not much more advanced a century later than this original theory of spinal degenerative processes.

However, this data is mostly observational data, and does not definitively prove how degeneration occurs. These mechanisms are complex. Many factors impact the rate and frequency of degeneration. Certain factors that are thought to impact the development of spinal degeneration are poorly understood, such as genetics. Although the basic cellular processes are not completely understood, a growing volume of medical research helps physicians understand what results in improved well-being for their patients.

5 Why Do I Both Have Neck and Arm Pain?

The cervical spine allows for us to turn our heads in relation to our body, and at the same time, protect our vital central nervous system. Generally speaking, the spinal cord is a bundle of nerves that sends signals to and from our brain to our body, allowing us to communicate with the outside enviroment. At each level of our cervical spine, a pair of spinal nerves exits in a region called the *neural foramen*. The region where the cervical spinal nerve exits, the neural foramen, is bordered by the disk space in front, a joint behind it, and bridges of bone above and below called *pedicles*. As you can see, the foramen is surrounded predominantly by bony structures with the exception of the disk space (Figure 5-1). The proximity of the disc space to the cervical nerve places one at risk from compression by disc herniation, as well as compression as the disk loses height during the process of disc degeneration. The narrowing of the foramen by any process is called *foraminal stenosis*.

Nerve Compression and Arm Pain

Compression of the nerve results in painful neck pain, often characterized by a sharp pain that radiates down the extremity. Depending on the level in the neck that the compression occurs, predictable patterns of radiating pain may occur. For example, at C4-C5, which describes the region between those two cervical levels where the C5 spinal nerve exits, pain often radiates down and terminates at the shoulder. At the C6 level pain often radiates downwards and terminates at the anterior upper arm and occasionally down to the thumb. At C7, patients often have pain radiating to the back of the arm terminating at the triceps and elbow, and occasionally radiating to the index and middle finger. At C8, patients most often have pain that radiates all the way down to the little finger (5th finger, 'pinkie') and adjacent half of the ring finger (4th finger from the thumb). These characteristic anatomic locations where sensation is provide by a specific nerve root are called dermatomes. **Variations in dermatomes exist, and this is thought to be explained by the variations between descriptions of the common dermatome patterns.**

Cervical Radiculopathy

Cervical radiculopathy is a medical condition marked by painful nerve root compression causing pain to radiate down the natural course of the nerve root, and result in variable sensory and motor symptoms supplied by that particular nerve root. It is a very common problem, and is thought to impact at least 83 per 100,000 people annually.[12] This pain is abrupt, sharp, and often, patients

---

12 *Radhakrishnan K, et al. Epidemiology of Cervical Radiculopathy. A population-based study from Rochester, Minnesota, 1976 through*

will characterize the pain as an 'electric shock'. The presence of severe, sharp pain, followed by painful sensory symptoms in the exact same location[13] (such as tingling) is a reliable symptom of cervical radiculopathy. However, depending on certain things usually determined in a patient's medical history, cervical radiculopathy becomes a more likely diagnosis. This can be accompanied by tingling in the same distribution as the radiating or lancinating pain. This pain is often followed by what is described as a goal painful ache, or a toothache. When the compression of the nerve is severe enough, this includes a degree of weakness.

Cervical radiculopathy is most often caused by nerve compression by a herniated cervical disc. The good news is, most patients will experience spontaneous improvement within the first three months of the onset of cervical radiculopathy caused by a herniated cervical disc. We will discuss treatment options for patients in the first several months including what treatment options that should be avoided earlier on, if at all possible. As a word of caution, there are always 'mimickers' that make the diagnosis of cervical radiculopathy more challenging. For example, degenerative shoulder conditions can overlap and the symptoms can occasionally be described as a radiating shoulder pain. Occasionally both symptoms are present.

How do I Interpret Foraminal Stenosis?

The degree, or severity of stenosis is the determining factor as to whether or not someone has symptoms from foraminal stenosis. A radiologist, a physician whose training is specifically in the skilled interpretation of imaging findings is the doctor who is responsible for writing your imaging reports that you bring to the doctor's office. Radiologists may grade stenosis by interpretation of your imaging-

---

1990. Brain. 1994;117(pt 2):325-335.

13 *Another term for the region of skin uniquely supplied by a nerve is called the dermatome.*

typically as mild, moderate, or the worst case, severe.

The Interpretation of Stenosis Varies

There are many systems for grading stenosis. There is no agreement as to the best method. While the practices of grading lumbar foraminal stenosis are more standardized, significant variations in nomenclature and technique can be found for cervical foraminal stenosis. The reason for this is is due to the anatomy. The lumbar foramen is larger and sagittal imaging provides a great view of the lumbar foramen, as it is perpendicular to the sagittal MRI slices. However, in contrast, cervical foramen are smaller and oriented at a 45-degree angle to the standard sagittal slices on an MRI, providing less than representative cross-sections. This anatomical difficulty has resulted in a significant variation in radiologist practice as to how stenosis is graded.

When interpreting stenosis, standardized grading systems are ideal because this leads to less confusion regarding the magnitude of the stenosis. Ideally, every radiologist, when given the same MRI, will conclude that there is the same degree of stenosis. However, in practice, there is variation, both among two different radiologists, and even variation when the same radiologists grade the same imaging at two different time points.[14] With that said, it is not uncommon for some radiologists to use the nonstandard terms 'mild-moderate' or 'moderate-severe' stenosis. Alternatively, other noncommittal modifiers have been encountered such as 'moderately mild' and 'moderately severe', which is not much different than the aforementioned hyphonated terms above. Unfortunately, either as a physician or a patient, it is impossible to tell what is

---

14 *Variability among two observers is called interobserver reliability and among the same radiologist at two different encounters with the same subject/study is called intraobserver reliability.*

meant from those terms.

Consistent grading is important, also because practices in imprecise grading decrease the significance of the reliance on grading in terms of medical decision making (Fig 5-1). On the other hand, higher grades correlate with the possibility that there will be neurologic manifestations (eg. weakness). Ideal grading systems are highly reliable and positively correlate with symptoms (higher grades are associated with more/worse symptoms)[15] important, as with other findings in spinal imaging, the extent of stenosis in many instances, the degree of foraminal stenosis is not always an indicator of a need for spinal surgery to decompress the nerve root.

Foraminal Stenosis: One Common Grading System

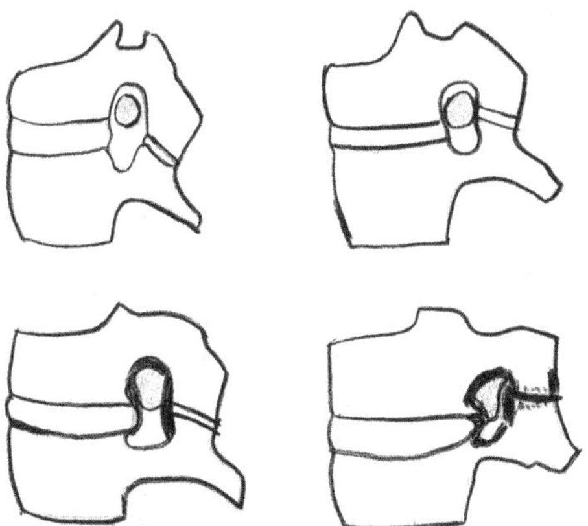

Figure 5 -1. Degrees of Foraminal Stenosis (simplified diagram): There are various scales for grading the degrees of stenosis. These all rely on spinal imaging. Typically, most neuroradiologist use an MRI to grade stenosis to the extent of nerve compression. Nerves can be visualized with an MRI and not with a CT. in patients that are unable to obtain an MRI, a CT myelogram is obtained (see imaging section regarding explanation of a CT mye-

---

15 *Park HJ et al. The clinical correlation of a new practical MRI method for grading cervical neural foraminal stenosis based on oblique sagittal images. AJR 203:412-417, 2014.*

logram). (Top left) this figure shows a cervical motion segment, which consists of 2 vertebrae and the intervening disc space. In the figure above, a side view is seen, where one can see the exiting nerve (shaded circle). There is a clear and continuous space between the nerve and the surrounding bone, which indicates that there is no foraminal stenosis (Top right). In this figure, you can see that there is a mild degree of stenosis, as you cannot see a continuous rim of space surrounding the nerve and there may be very minimal nerve compression. (Bottom left) With spondylosis, one begins to observe on imaging an enlargement of the bone adjacent to the discs as well as the joints on the opposite side of the nerve as well. This results in nerve compression. In moderate stenosis seen here, there is compression of the nerve which amounts to less than 50% narrowing of that foramen. (Bottom right) in severe stenosis there is greater than 50% narrowing of the neuroforamen and substantial nerve root compression which may be equal to or greater than 50% of the diameter of the nerve. These nuances and the extent of foraminal narrowing and nerve root compression is varied by the type of imaging sequence used and technique. Some of these techniques have variability among examiners/radiologist. However, across these studies, worsening stenosis on imaging correlates with a greater likelihood of having symptoms attributable to that compression.

6 What Are the Common Soft Tissue Injuries That Cause Neck Pain?

The neck is the most mobile part of the spine, providing the greatest range of motion of any part of the spine. Numerous muscles and ligaments support our neck alignment and provide for conditions that allow for these motions to occur while protecting the nerves that enter and exit the cervical spine. There are so many muscular and ligamentous attachments. In fact, they are impossible to distinguish on our most advanced imaging, the MRI. Due to our reliance on our spinal muscles on a daily basis, injured muscle is increasingly relied upon and not afforded the adequate time for recovery. This can cause chronic ligamentous or muscular injury and ultimately a pattern of chronic neck pain. Muscle strain is undoubtably the most common cause of neck pain. Muscles and tendons in the back can easily become overloaded and cause neck and LBP. This type of pain will go away with rest, but this does not mean the avoidance of activity. Muscle strain that is particularly intense, and in older patients, can take relatively longer time periods to heal (months).

When more serious muscular injury occurs, shortening or scarring of the muscle can occur, which is manifested by firm, tender, nodules in the large muscles groups of the neck and shoulder girdle (Fig. 6-1). Is this the explanation for every firm, tender nodule? Due to the many medical causes of a new mass (including the less common, such as cancer) that can be felt underneath the skin, it is especially important that you show this to your healthcare provider. In the majority of cases where nodules are associated with recent strenuous activity, trigger point injections are a very helpful option.

Trigger Point Injections

Muscle strain can be relieved by trigger point injections. The muscle is primarily inflamed and most often relieves with injections of anti-inflammatory medications (most often using a steroid such as cortisol or triamcinolone, or along with another non-steroidal anti-inflammatory medication). Beyond that, the pathophysiology (ie. speicific scientific explanation) is fairly unclear related to trigger points, despite success with trigger point injections at relieving pain in the ambulatory and emergency room setting.[16] Trigger point injections are not tolerated universally. Citing data from one randomized controlled trial, lidocaine patches are effective equivalent options, which are patches that effectively numb the skin in the trigger point region.[17]

---

16 *Wong CS et al. A New Look at Trigger Point Injections. Anesthesiol Res PRact. 2012.*

17 *Affaitati G et al. A randomized, controlled study comparing a lidocaine patch, a placebo patch, and anesthetic injection for treatment of*

Muscle Strain, Trigger Points, And Nodules

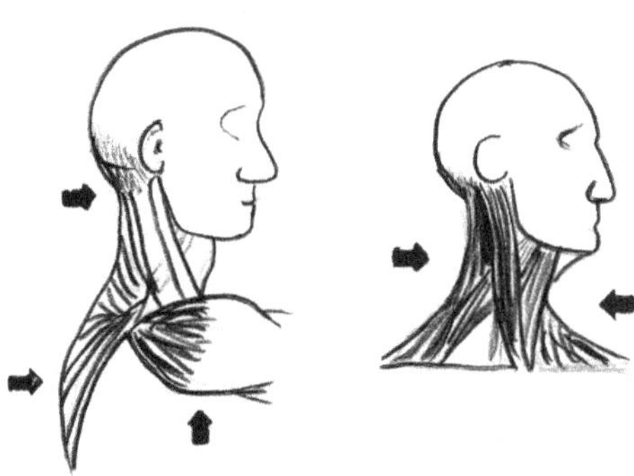

Figure 6-1. Trigger Points are pain generators located in muscle under constant tension. Often, areas can contract and become inflamed, resulting in nodules that can be felt underneath the skin, which are muscular contracations.

These injections do not require x-ray guidance as with the spinal injections, and are not specific to any problem on an MRI, and are therefore unrelated to a specific level of the lumbar spine. As a reminder, pain centered over the neck is never an indicator of a spinal source of pain, or any structure in general such as the clavicle or scapula. It is more or less, a starting point for diagnosis and treatment. So, pain from a cervical or cervicothoracic disc (region at bottom of cervical spine near the top of the thoracic spine) can give the sense of generalized neck pain. **Most commonly, generalized neck pain originates in the muscles on the back of the neck and does not improve without allowing adequate**

---

trigger points in patients with myofascial pain syndrome: evaluation of pain and somatic pain thresholds.

time for recovery, which includes strict avoidance of all exacerbating activities.

Musculoskeletal Inflammation: 'Overworked' Muscles Are The Most Common Generator of Neck Pain

Throughout the spine, regardless of region, most of muscles that attach to the bone via tendons and allow for movement and provide posture are located posterior (behind) the spine. The most common cause of neck pain due to inflammation in the muscles and soft tissue of the neck occurs posterior to the spine. The normal cervical spine is lordotic, matching the curvature of the lumbar spine (the neck is 'arched', like the low back) as with most people with normal spinal alignment, and opposes the curvature of the thoracic spine which is referred to as kyphosis ('hunchback' is a term nobody uses in healthcare but paints a clear image of what an exaggerated kyphotic posture looks like).

Imaging of the Cervical Spine: An Increasingly More Common Tool That is Not Diagnostic for Axial Neck Pain

Sometimes there is a correlation between painful symptoms and diseases, such as a disc herniation occuring on the same side (eg. disc herniation on the right side with right-sided neck pain). However, just because this correlation is found, does not mean that one has identified the problem. Statistically, this simultaneous occurance is common because pre-existing spinal degeneration is ongoing, and a naturally occuring process in all people, prior to eventually having symptoms. **It is an eventuality that everyone will have spinal symptoms related to degeneration. For that reason, the presence of same-sided axial back**

pain and degenerative spinal conditions on an MRI is not conclusive evidence that the cause of the pain has been identified. It is even less likely that one's neck pain is due to a spinal problem occuring on the opposite side of one's symptoms, although, with general (axial) neck pain **without radicular pain (see, arm and neck pain)** some overlap can occur. Therefore, correlating generalized neck symptoms to spinal degeneration is less helpful. Moreover, this is part of the reason for the mixed degrees of success in treating generalized back and neck pain with both surgical and nonsurgical means (some may argue that the main reason for this is that the workup is far more extensive than common practice, but this claim cannot be substantiated without an organized study that provides a 'far more extensive' workup). In summary, neck pain is not unlike its low back pain counterpart, and should be viewed as a nonspecific symptom.

Opposing Groups of Neck Muscles Aid in Complex Motions and Help Balance The Head and Neck

The **extensor muscles** are broken into two groups, capital extensors and cervical extensors. Capital extensors attach to the skull and are important for extending the neck (moving the head backwards, as in to look upwards), while cervical extensors support the posture of the neck. Without cervical extensors, and in extreme examples of this where these muscles do not function appropriately, a 'chin-on-chest' deformity can occur (Fig. 6-2).

The **flexor muscles** are the muscular attachments to the front of the spine, cervical flexors are far less developed. Capital flexors are much fewer, and are vital for allowing the head to bend forward, to lower the chin, or to look downwards. Since gravity assists with this, in part due to the way our spine is balanced (in a manner that the center of gravity is over our pelvis and feet), these muscles are much less developed. There are also cervical flexors, and they have a minimal contribution to the movements of the neck. However, they can be initially referred to as accessory respiratory muscles, meaning, they can support your diaphragm in respiration.

Contraction And Shortening Of Unopposed Muscle Groups Result In Neck Flexion and Extension

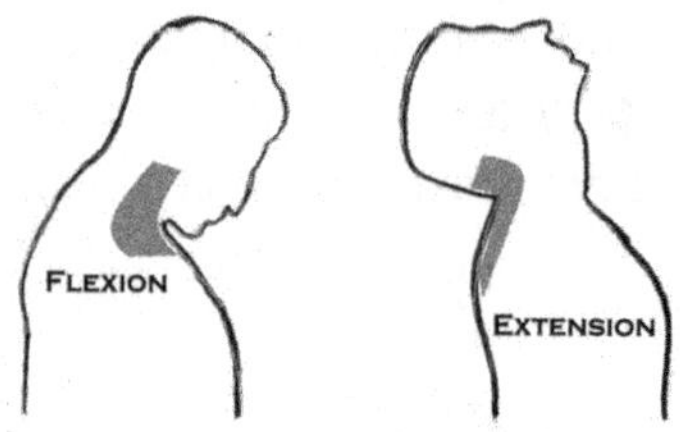

Figure 6-2. Neck Extension is facilitated by posterior musculature, which upon activation results in contraction and shortening of the muscle, which then pulls the posterior skull (occiput) and spine backwards, resulting in extension (right image, muscles are shaded). Opposing this action is neck flexion, which similarly results in shortening of musculature in predominantly anterior muscle groups. These muscle groups are far less developed, and flexion is assisted by gravity (left image).

Common Causes of Neck Pain Related To Spinal Degeneration

Discogenic Pain	painful disc degeneration/ inflammation involving the disc and adjacent bone.
Myofascial Pain	muscle strain (ligamentous sprain is uncommon and prompt requires evaluation).
Facet Joint Pain	Athritis of the paired joints of a spinal level. For every disc, there are a right and left-sided facet joint.
Spinal Stenosis with Cervical Myelopathy	Symptomatic compression of the spinal cord in the central spinal canal which may cause difficulty walking, sensory distburbances in the arms and legs, extremity pain, weakness, clumsiness in the hands, and eventual bowel and bladder disturbances can occur.

7 What Is the Most Common Cause of Neck Pain?

Neck pain is complex, and can often have multiple causes. The most common causes is muscle strain. While the majority of complaints are thought to be muscular, damage to any of the numerous superficial and deep structures in the neck and the base of the skull as well as the upper thorax and shoulder girdle can be perceived as neck pain (Fig. 7-1).[18] There is tremendous overlap in pain re-

18 *Shoulder girdle: Collectively, the musculoskeletal structures allowing for upper limb limb movement. The trapezius, rhomboids, serratus anterior, pectoralis minor, and levator scapulae attach to the clavicle and scapula allowing for motion at 3 major joints.*

ferral[19], as the source of the pain is not adjacent to the area of pain. It is not always realistic to self-diagnose given these complexities; In other words, seeking professional help may be necessary to help identify the cause of the problem. Prior to that appointment, keep track of the specific symptoms, how long they last, how frequent, any other associated symptoms, factors that provoke the pain, and provide relief. Often a journal may be necessary if this is a chronic problem. **A physician will often ask about associated weakness, arm pain, or sensory symptoms in the region of the pain. Also, pain when you sneeze, or pain provoked by any kind of neck movement. Keep in mind, red flag symptoms prompt urgent attention (see section, red flag symptoms).**

Neck Pain Driven By Muscle Spasms Involves Many Muscle Groups

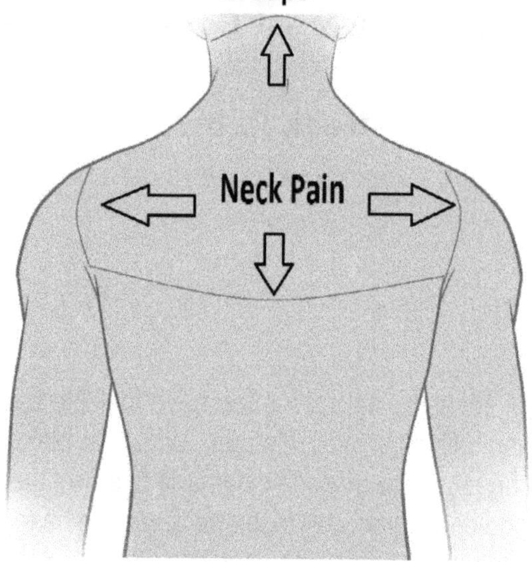

Figure 7-1. Neck Pain. Neck pain driven by spinal musculature is not just

19 *Referred pain: pain felt in one location, which is different than the origin of the source of pain. Eg. Some kidney and abdominal aortic diseases can cause lumbar pain.*

limited to paraspinal muscles. Muscle groups and their attachments to the thoracic spine, clavicle, scapula, shoulder, sternum, and skull can become inflamed and cause neck pain. Muscle inflammation can be relieved by oral anti-inflammatory medications and even injections. However, the treatment process for any inflammation should begin with a thorough process of identifying the underlying cause of inflammation.

Key Points

- Neck pain flare-ups are most often musculoskeletal, originating from one of the many small muscles that attach to the bones of the spine, shoulder, clavicle, sternum, and scapula. There are numerous small muscles, ligaments, tendons, and fascia (connective tissue) that supports the alignment of the spine.

- These structures are subjected to constant daily stress, facilitated by poor ergonomics such as chronic neck flexion for cell phone use. Overuse of specific muscles causes acute muscle strain, which ranges from muscular stretch injuries to complete tears. Sprains involve stretch or tear injuries to the ligaments. Ligaments in the neck and back are very tough, designed to withstand a high degree of force prior to failure (complete disruption), and will not completely tear, except in the case of major trauma, or rarely, a ligament can harden (*ossification*)[20]. Strains and sprains are usually a source of

---

20 *Ossification of the Posterior Longitudinal Ligament (OPLL) is a condition seen less commonly in the United States than Asia, where the ligament behind the posterior vertebral bodies, the posterior longitudinal lig-*

chronic back pain and are the focus of many non-invasive back pain treatments, including stretching, physical therapy, and chiropracter treatment.

- Appropriate posture is essential in preventing neck pain. Workplace ergonomics is something to consider (see chapter, *ergonomics*). If you have a computer at work- just remember, your desk and chair are adjustable. Most importantly, the neck and upper back should not be doing exaggerated compensation- the equipment around you should be. This leads to unnatural neck positioning, loading of certain muscles, and finally, a risk of chronic neck pain.

- An imaging study will 'find' a condition of the spine. A finding of a spinal degenerative disease doesn't necessarily cause symptoms. This is where a spinal expert can help you go through the diagnostic process and guide you along the road to getting better. For example, 'having a spur' is common and does not carry any meaning by itself (see imaging section regarding 'spurs' and other imaging findings). **There is a reason why it is called a finding, because no cause-and-effect relationship is established yet, merely by looking at a picture.**

---

ament, calcifies and hardens over time. This predisposes the neck to fractures, and more commonly, to advanced stenosis due to the growth of calcium deposits that eventually can fill the spinal canal and cause symptomatic spinal cord compression. However, most people with OPLL are thought to be asymptomatic.

Spinal Causes of Neck Pain

There are numerous causes of spinal pain, and a comprehensive list of diagnoses can be found in a multi-volume spinal textbook. In fact, physicians are taught to obtain a careful history and physical examination, and to mentally consider potential diagnostic categories before reviewing specific diagnoses. Even the list of categories is fairly extensive and includes traumatic, infectious, vascular, autoimmune, metabolic, neoplastic,congenital, iatrogenic, degenerative, endocrine, social, and even behavioral!

Fortunately, experience helps the physician quickly achieve a diagnosis without having to independently persue these many rabbit holes with time consuming and fruitless tests and studies. By far, the most common causes of cervical spinal pain is muscular, and this is similar to low back pain. Additionally, chronic low back pain can cause neck pain due to postural changes and muscle activation! The two groups work in tandem to achieve a neutral 'global' spinal alignment. However, paraspinal muscle spasms may just be one manifestation of the second most common cause, which is a spinal degenerative process, such as cervical degenerative disc disease.

Disc Degeneration Affects Multiple Levels At Varying Rates

Degeneration of the disk is more common at the C5-6 and C6-7 levels because they receive greater forces from the levels above.[21] They are also at that point of transition from the flexible cervical

---

21 *One analogy for this would be the 'low man on the totem pole' analogy where the lower discs of the cervical and lumbar spine carry the weight of the men above.*

spine to the stiffer thoracic spine. The thoracic spine is not very flexible and is stabilized by the ribs as well. This extra stabilization, and the lack of mechanical range of motion is thought to result in the lower rate of disc degeneration and least contribution to spinal pain. The transition zone of the flexible cervical spine to the stiffer thoracic spine, puts increased wear and tear in this region.

Acitivies that cause chronic neck flexion, such as texting, are thought to load the cervical-thoracic transition zone and cause increased disc pressure, pressure on the facet joints, and muscle pain at the C5-6 and C6-7 levels (see section on text neck).

Depression, Neck Pain, and Pain Processing

Chronic pain can cause depression and anxiety, which usually takes greater than 3 months to occur.[22] Also, depression most often manifests itself with physical symptoms first and foremost. Of a large study of 1146 patients diagnosed with depression, 69% of them reported only physical symptoms as their reasons to come to the outpatient clinic.[23] It is very difficult to remain objective and to know which occurred first. However, experienced clinicians are available and willing to help.

Depression has numerous studied effects. It impacts natural steroid production, which are anti-inflammatory chemicals. Having lowered natural anti-inflammatory chemicals in the body may lead to increased pain. Also, pain signal processing is impacted, which can increase someone's sensitivity to less painful stimuli pain, as

---

22 *Schofferman, Jerome M.D. in, What to do for a pain in the neck: the complete program for neck pain relief, pp. 256-274.*

23 *Simon GE et al. An international study of the relation between somatic symptoms and depression. N Engl J Med. 341:658-659, 1999.*

well as having a lower pain tolerance. Overall, these are just theories, and have been very difficult to prove. Moreover, psychological stress in our lives, anxiety-provoking events, personal loss, major depression, and posttraumatic stress disorder all influence pain processing. Counseling is often necessary to identify the underlying drivers psychosomatic pain, which is physical pain driven by stress, anxiety, or other conscious social, behavioral, or psychological factor.

Depression and the Neurotransmitter

The link between depression and neck and back pain is more likely explained by a chemical imbalance in the absence of other physical (somatic) explanations (eg. fracture, severe stenosis, etc...). A deficiency in norepinephrine, as well as serotonin, found in depression, is thought to decrease pain tolerance.[24] Depression is therefore treated medically to correct neurotransmitter imbalances with selective norepinephrine reuptake inhibitors (SNRIs) and selective serotonine reuptake inhibitors (SSRIs). Another class of antidepressants, the tricyclic antidepressants (TCSAs), such as nortryptyline, amitryptyline, and desipramine may be relatively more effective at improving the painful symptoms. These are much more generally researched for low back pain than neck pain, and the overall research quality is low. [25] Again, in medicine, when research quality is low, there will always be groups of physicians favoring different protocols for treatment. And these healthcare professionals have your best interest in mind and their unique experience may lend them to suggest a particular treatment.

---

24 *Jaracz J et al Unexplained painful physical symptoms in patients with major depressive disorder: prevalence, pathophysiology and management. CNS Drugs 2016 30:29-304, 2016.*

25 *Urquhart DM et al. Efficacy of low-dose amitriptyline for chronic low back pain: a randomized clinical trial. JAMA Intern med, 178(11): 2018.*

If doctors cannot agree on the connection between depression and back and neck pain, there is one thing that most people cannot dispute: Depression decreases the likelihood of a successful treatment. People with depression have the lowest satisfaction scores on any kind of backpain treatment, surgical or nonsurgical. Duloxetine is a class of antidepressant that can modulate the levels of serotonin and norepinephrine in the body. It is also been shown to be helpful when given for the relief of back and neck pain, although there are severeal high-quality randomized trials showing the relief of chronic low back pain with duloxetine, leading to FDA approval for chronic low back pain and musculoskeletal pain. While the mechanism of how duloxetine treats chronic pain is not entirely understood, the key point is that spinal pain treatment is often multimodal (utilizing more than one class of medication - eg. muscle relaxant plus an anti-inflammatory, etc..). Subsequent sections address common questions that pertain to cervical spinal surgery in patients with depression. In general, untreated depression is a negative predictor of success.

Posture and Neck Pain

Neck pain can often be explained in many instances by a postural explanation - i.e. neck pain is caused by poor posture. This is different than compensation for spinal alignment, which is a separate and complexed discussion that eludes even some very experienced specialists. The theory of a postural cause suggests a cause-and-effect relationship between poor shoulder posture placing undue stress to the muscles and ligaments of the neck which causes chronic neck pain. This has fallen out of favor as a general explanation for chronic neck pain, it is again a very difficult concept to prove or disprove. However, this concept prevails in the workplace as poor workplace ergonomics results in chronic poor posture, for the majority of each day, and is functionally similar.

Chronic Neck Pain May Have Numerous Causes

More than likely, in the author's opinion, most people have general, chronic neck pain as a result of numerous stressors. A few examples include excessive physical activity at the workplace or with exercise, resulting in chronic muscular strain. Numerous causes of neck pain are often present, all contributing to the general problem: an insufficient recovery period, suboptimal ergonomics (eg. a television or monitor mounted too high, eg. well above a horizontal gaze, resutling in prolonged extension of the neck), poor posture, and even depression.

SECTION II

ACUTE NECK PAIN MANAGEMENT

8 Cervical Red Flags: When Should I Seek Help For Neck Pain?

Abrupt, severe neck or back pain can be debilitating and scary. Often, when patients call for advice they are sent to the nearest emergency department, which can add fear and anxiety to the pain. **While most episodes of severe acute neck pain will resolve spontaneously without requiring any treatment, is common for patients to receive a wide variety of treatments and diagnostic tests earlier on.** Part of the reason for this is because of the lack of a standardized protocol for neck pain management. There are many reasons why practitioners vary in terms of management of acute neck pain. A few of the main reasons are discussed below.

There Are No Standardized Protocols For Management

- **Generalized Neck Pain Is Non-specific:** Finding a definitive diagnosis of neck pain is very difficult (see *causes of neck pain*). As a result, neck pain management varies. There is a wide spectrum of underlying spinal diseases, some of which are very disabling.
- **Lack of a Standardized Protocol:** There is no standard-

ized protocol for workup of neck pain. Protocols have been recommended by general medical societies, but in the absence of high-quality research studies that test care algorithms, changes have been mainly implemented by insurance companies. To some extent, when an insurance company denies coverage for an MRI, this is not universally to one's detriment if that person experiences spontaneous improvement while awaiting the outcome of an authorization.

- **Medicolegal**: Neck pain and back pain as they pertain to the workplace and personal injury, as well as the fear of the provider to reach a timely diagnosis are just a few of the issues that sway a healthcare provider towards obtaining an early MRI (<3 months).

- **Consumerism In Healthcare:** Due to increased costs of care (partly due to the above), value-based care metrics are being implemented. A value-based care metric is a measure of a quality-of-life improvement, instead of quantity (eg. payment for number of surgeries). On the surface, the goal is to decrease the volume of treatments where the benefits are minimal, and the net result of this will be that less money is spent on healthcare services. The services that are being performed where patients get the least benefit will be paid the least amount of money, which will be measured in a satisfaction survey. As a result, one unintended concern of this change in the marketplace is that a physician will be less willing to refuse unnecessary tests and treatments to patients, out of a concern that their pay will be linked to patient satisfaction, in effect transforming the care dynamics to one seen in a standard business, where "the customer is always right." Regardless of who is right regarding this debate, this is one additional reason why one may get an earlier MRI.

Cervical Red Flags

The majority of medical problems are related to common degenerative conditions of the spine both in the low back and neck. **However, some conditions warrant early medical attention.** While there is no definite rule encompassing all scenarios, there are a number of general findings either from past medical, surgical, social history, and symptoms of yours that may constitute a "Red Flag Conditions". 'Red flags' can be physical exam findings, signs (detected by the physican), or symptoms, or a specific past medical history where low back pain may raise concern (hence, red flags) for a serious condition.

There is some debate over the ability of these 'red flags' to predict an underlying medical process is going on apart from a muscle sprain or disc herniation. However, these 'red flags' included in the table are troubling and require an urgent evaluation from a health-care provider. The following table contains a summary of 'red flags' published by the American College of Physicians and the American Pain Society. One example would be someone with a history of cancer and back pain, which could be a sign of cancer involvement of the spine. Another example would be someone with a depressed immune system, and the recentonset of new back pain symptoms and fevers. This combination of symptoms may be a sign of a spinal infection. Delay in diagnosis and treatment for these medical conditions can lead to worsening spinal involvement and likely a greater risk to the patient.

Neck Pain Red Flags: Key Points

The American College of Physicians has guidelines proposed

specifically for low back pain. These can be broadly applied to the neck in many instances. However, if at any time one's symptoms are severe or concerning enough, it is appropriate to seek medical attention.

- Previous history of cancer and/or, elevated markers of inflammation (ESR. CBC), or weight loss

- History of cancer: In the case of a cancer history, severe neck pain or new neurologic symptoms could be a worrisome sign ranging from a mild reaction to prescribed medications, or even so far as to indicate possible spread of cancer to the spine. In this case, always discuss new symptoms with your physician or care team.

- Neck pain and fevers: These are a concerning combination of symptoms which could herald a spinal or neighboring soft tissue infection. Cervical spinal infections can be life threatening, and are often seen with intravenous drug abuse. Fever and back pain is especially worrisome in patients taking antibiotics for active or chronic infections, immunocompromised patients (weak immune system), and patients with prior spinal surgery and neighboring back pain.

- Concern for cauda equina syndrome: Cauda new urinary retention, incontinence, back pain, and/or changes of sensation in the groin/perianal area(numbness)

- Prior spinal surgery

- Known spinal condition AND new or worsening symptoms

Cervical Spine 'Red Flags' Requiring Urgent Medical Attention

▪ Severe Neck Pain with a History of Cancer
▪ Intravenous drug/recreational drug Abuse
▪ Weight loss

▪ Hoarseness, Trouble Swallowing, Neck Fullness
▪ Fevers
▪ Bowel or Bladder Incontinence/Dysfunction
▪ Trouble Walking/Balance Problems
▪ Muscle Weakness
▪ Loss of Hand Functioning/Dexterity
▪ Other Associated Neurologic Symptoms
▪ Above Symptoms or Unrelenting Pain with a History of Prior Cervical Spine Surgery

9 What Can I Do Immediately For Neck Pain?

Severe, sharp neck pain due to a disc herniation can be very debilitating. **If your symptoms are limited to pain and some sensory symptoms such as tingling or burning in the same region, most people will experience improvement without any treatment, whatsoever.**

Do I Need To Go To The Emergency Room?

A trip to the emergency department is most often unnecessary. This problem is very expensive for our society as a whole, and delays access of patients that require these specialized resources. Healthcare institutions are increasing the pathways to allow for people with acute neck and low back pain to get urgent medical attention to those who need it, in an increasing number of venues. This book will focus on a few of the many specific alternatives to the emergency room including the primary care practice, urgent care center, and a few other popular locations including pain management practices and the chiropractic practice.

Do I Need Immediate Imaging of My Neck?

Many societies recommend avoiding any imaging such as a Cervical MRI, Cervical CT, or Cervical X-Ray for the first 3 months, if at all possible. A CT or X-ray is not sufficient to detect nerve root or spinal cord compression. While disc herniations may occasionally be seen on a CT, most people have evidence of some type of a disc herniation with or without any neck pain, and therefore not a diagnosis of the underlying cause of pain. The nerve roots do not show up on a CT and an MRI is needed to diagnose nerve root compression. However, we will discuss imaging in detail in the following imaging section.

One final consideration is that once someone has their first MRI, it is more than likely that they have committed themselves to accepting that some aspect of the degenerative spinal conditions are contributing to their pain and therefore they need to treat that identified spinal issue. This leads to more treatments, prescriptions, referrals, follow up imaging, and often, surgery.

Why Would Medical Societies Guide Physicians to Avoid Invasive Treatments, Opiate Use, and Advanced Imaging in the First 3 Months?

For the reasons above, many patients are able to avoid the long journey of going through the spinal pain treatment pathway by avoiding imaging and aggressive pain treatments their first 3 months. Just as with low back pain, abrupt onset neck or neck and arm pain improves, regardless of the intervention over the first 3 months.

Opiate addiction has been compared to the HIV epidemic, in the scale of the number of deaths attributed to addiction. In the last several years, federal and state legislation have completely changed the way that addictive analgesic medications (pain meds) are prescribed, with the goal to limit drug dependence and major complications, such as the death. All medical societies have urged providers to limit prescribing of controlled substances and especially to avoid potentially harmful medications(such as addictive opiate medications) and other invasive treatments.

Summary of American College of Physicians General Recommendations for Neck Pain (2017)

- In the 2017 guidelines by the American College of Physicians: physicians are urged to avoid prescribing medications for acute low back pain (<4 weeks), which can include opioids, steroids, tricyclic antidepressants, and selective serotonin reuptake inhibitors (SSRIs).
- Often the pain is very severe limited most daily activity. If patients see their doctor, it would be preferred to start with a nonsteroidal anti-inflammatory drugs (NSAIDS) or skeletal muscle relaxants.
- Also, within the first four weeks, massage, acupuncture, or spinal manipulation therapy(chiropracters) are reasonable options for pain relief.
- After 12 weeks, pharmacotherapy with nonsteroidal anti-inflammatory drugs, tramadol, or duloxetine is reasonable. Tramadol is a controlled substance and is addicting.
- Opioids are only an option if these other medications have

failed. These are a last resort medication.

10 Where Can I Get Help, and Where is

the First Place To Go?

If one does not have any red flag symptoms, then the best place to go would be scheduling an urgent appointment with a **primary care provider/physician's office**. While it is common to have acute neck pain of sudden onset, it is uncommon for one to be harboring a diagnosis that requires emergent treatment. **Another consideration would be urgent care.** Should one arrive after normal hours, an urgent care center may be a better option than a hospital. Wait times are impacted by many issues that are specific to one's circumstances, such as availability and wait times to get an MRI and in more densely populated areas one would expect to wait longer. However, a trip to the urgent care center is significantly less expensive.

For more detail regarding red flag symptoms, refer to the previous chapter discussing associated symptoms of neck and back pain that require urgent work-up (red flags).

What Are The Centers Specializing In Neck Pain Relief?[26]

- Primary Care Clinic

---

26 *Take note that that the best route is often to seek care from someone who is familiar with your medical history, and that you have an established relationship with, which is traditionally at your primary care practicioner's office. However, other options are available if this is not always possible. This list is not comprehensive. Prior to an appointment ask the clinic of interest about all treatments available, before finding out after 2 months that a needed treatment is not available.*

- Pain Management Practice
- Neurosurgery and Orthopedic Clinics
- Neurology Clinics
- Urgent Care
- Emergency Department
- Chiropractic Center

Scheduling and External Forces Directing Care

For neck pain without red flag symptoms, there are many places where appropriate care can be obtained and are listed on the previous page. In many communities the choice of where to go is often dictated by expertise and availability- this often takes the difficult decision of where and when to go out of one's hands. That can be helpful in the case of a nonurgent appointment, but less so in the case of an urgent pain issue. Ultimately, if the duration of time to get an appointment is too long, then visits such as urgent care and emergency room visits are certainly options.

Spine Surgeon Availability And The Growing US Population

Often, patients would like to be referred directly to a spine surgeon for evaluation. While neurological and orthopedic surgery clinics are seeing more patients with acute neck and back pain, wait time is growing in some high population density areas. This is because of the tremendous growth in population that is not matched with specialty surgical services. Anecdotally, in 1977, the government-funded Study on Surgical Services for the United States (SOSSUS) published recommendations that an ideal ratio be met of no less than 1 neurosurgeon per 100,000.[27] However, a multifaceted analysis shows numerous indicators that the needs are not being met and the situation is not improving— these include factors such as the rate of growth and average age of our US population, the overall workforce and average age of the neurosurgeon, the average number of neurosurgeon job vacancies, the numerous obstacles to training larger numbers of neurosurgery residents, the declining trauma neurosurgeon coverage, and so on.[28] Returning to patient needs with regards to acute neck pain care, in some parts of the US a 3-4 month wait for a spine evaluation for acute neck pain care seems unrealistic. Therefore, an open mind is needed with regards to the many acceptable and excellent alternatives to one's preferred neck pain care.

---

27 *Zuidema GD. The SOSSUS report and its impact on neurosurgery. J Neurosurg. 1977;46(2):135-144*

28 *Statement of the American Association of Neurological Surgeons American Board of Neurological Surgery Congress of Neurological Surgeons, and Society of Neurological Surgeons before the Institute of Medicine On The Subject of Ensuring An Adequate Neurosurgical Workforce For the 21st Century. published December 19, 2012 in https://www.aans.org/pdf/Legislative/Neurosurgery%20IOM%20GME%20Paper%2012%2019%2012.pdf*

The Convenience Of Integrated Care

However, some locations are more efficient than others. One example is the so-called comprehensive clinic. The term 'comprehensive' is frequently used in orthopedic and other pain clinics to indicate that this location contains most, if not, many of the necessary diagnostic and treatment components all in one location. For example, many 'comprehensive' spine clinics advertise a prompt same-day evaluation and the ability to obtain a prompt assessment, workup including CT and MRI, even imaging preliminary interpretation, and treatment. These centers are able to provide this because all of the components are there at one clinic, including all treatment options, diagnostic imaging facilities, physical therapists, a pharmacy, and even pain management specialist and surgeon. The question of efficiency becomes clear in our minds when one has had the fortune and convenience of having every aspect of a medical issue managed in one integrated healthcare facility. Now, contrast this with multiple appointments at geographically isolated facilities, all in different heatlhcare systems or private offices, with these several appointments spaced out weeks at a time.

Potential Drawback of Highly Efficient Systems

Efficiency may not always be the most helpful for uncomplicated neck pain, as some highly efficient algorithms for care include rapid acquisition of imaging studies and several evaluations. Opponents to this system are usually payers, but in addition many include some primary care medical societies. Opponents to early imaging argue that the pain most often resolves spontaneously, and secondarily, imaging studies are driving up the cost of low back pain care. After all, total direct costs to US healthcare was estimated at over 85 billion US Dollars in 2005 for managing low back pain.[29] Many healthcare experts argue that advanced imaging is usually not necessary if the pain improves spontaneously in the majority of patients.

Indeed, most flare-ups of axial neck pain decline substantially in the *first month* according to large study.[30] **In another review of the literature, the natural course is summarized: "Acute neck pain resolves within days or weeks, but may become chronic in about 10% of people."**[31] This argues that there is little need for imaging and other 'advanced' or 'invasive' treatments in most patients with acute neck pain without red flag symptoms. Many insurance companies are familiar with this, and require a physical therapy program for a variable duration of 8-12 weeks prior to authorizing an MRI. This is more of a strategy to avoid the expense of advanced patient imaging. that ultimately have spontaneous neck pain relief. to see if the pain resolves before they find themselves getting many kinds of advanced treatment options, such as epidural and facet injections.

Sometimes waiting to see if symptoms improve is not always an option, especially if it worsens. Trained staff members at emergency department and urgent care facilities are able to be seen and provide either reassurance or further needed workup that cannot wait. However, seeing emergency healthcare staff for neck pain without radiation down the extremity, neurologic symptoms, and without any complicating factors (see chapter on *red flags*) usually results in a short term temporizing measures being taken.

---

29 *Martin BI, et al. Expenditures and health status among adults with back and neck problems. JAMA. 299(6)656-64: 2008.*

30 *Vasseljen O et al. Natural course of acute neck and low back pain in the general population. Pain. 154(8)1237-1244:2013.*

31 *Binder AI. Neck Pain, BMJ Clin Evid. 2008:1103.*

Summary

In summary, most flare-ups of neck pain resolve spontaneously, and in line with the 2017 guidelines by the American College of Physicians (ACP), the most conservative approach is always favored, which is avoidance of activies that exacerbate the pain, over the counter analgesics, observation, and physical therapy. The best starting point is usually with the one most familiar with your care, which in most cases is your personal physician. This is usually a primary care clinic, but is many settings it is a number of facilities. If there are any questions as to the urgency of someone's symptoms, then refer to the section, Red Flags, or the following section that discusses urgency.

More options have been added in the last decade to address the growth and age of our population seeking care for spinal degenerative conditions. In general, the likelihood you will encounter some of these large, 'comprehensive' practices depends on the region that you live. Typically, this is seen in populations requiring a growing number of options to keep up with the demand. Lastly, for the reasons above, and for the reason of the large demand and limited supply, many care pathways for neck pain will almost feel automated or, 'beyond our control'. At times like this, read through the sections of this book and realize that if one knows exactly where to look, numerous options are available.

11 What Are Some Of The Distinguishing Features of A Primary Care, Urgent Care, The Pain Clinic, And The Emergency Department?

If one is unable to get an appointment to see a primary care physician, there are many alternatives in the modern healthcare setting. At the very least, these options can help you obtain some pain relief while you wait for your appointment. This chapter will help address these options in 2020. As you read each section below, you will be surprised by the number of options. To help you organize them, the first and most important question that must be answered before proceeding assess the urgent nature of the neck pain. It is important to assess whether there are any associated neurological symptoms, or are there any of the red flag symptoms/medical history?[32] If it is just predominantly neck pain, then the next most important questions is, "Can medical attention wait until normal business hours?" This is typically eight in the morning until 5 in the afternoon. This separates the treatment options into manageable groups from there one. Further questions then help you sort out the differences between some locations.

---

32 *The most relevent associated neurological symptoms with neck pain include numbness, tingling, weakness, loss of grip and dexterity in the hands, inability to walk, and bowel and bladder symptoms. Please refer to the table on chapter 8 for a list of red flag symptoms.*

Are There Any Additional Neurological And/Or Red Flag Symptoms?

Neurologic Symptoms, or 'red flags' require urgent attention at the nearest emergency department, or potentially an urgent care center. While there are many other clinics that provide neck and low back pain treatment, the capabilities vary. In general, should one have neurological symptoms in addition to neck pain, or red flag symptoms, the most appropriate place to go would be to the emergency department so that one can get an immediate evaluation. This is even more valid should one be experiencing a decline in strength, sensation, ability to walk, or loss of bowel or bladder sensation. This is considered an emergency. While this is the most common recommendation, and remains to be the policy at many centers, some facilities are able to arrange for a patient to urgently obtain an MRI through an outpatient clinic, in an attempt to decrease wait times at emergency departments. These capabilities vary and this would be something that you would have to have firsthand knowledge of or be able to inquire about in a timely manner before making an urgent appointment. If one chooses to go to an outpatient clinic, that person would have to make an appointment with a provider and they would have to order an MRI and they can obtain an MRI potentially at that facility or clinic, provided this is available. Otherwise, that person would have to be sent to another clinic to get an MRI urgently and then, the expectation would be that that person would have someone who can have that MRI interpretted shortly after, and then recommendations be made shortly following the MRI acquisition. An urgent care center is more likely able to do this then an outpatient primary care facility or spine specialist office, which generally is limited in the scope of practice and certainly the practice is limited by usual operating business hours, i.e., 8 a.m. or 9 a.m. to 5 p.m.

Can I Wait Until Normal Daytime Hours?

This is a question that only the patient can answer. Pain relief and pain tolerance can only be assessed on an individual basis. The following options may be considered in the event of severe pain:

- Urgent Care Clinic
- Emergency Department (24 hours)
- Specialty Spinal Care (orthopedic and neurosurgery clinics/pain management)[33]

Another consideration, should you have intractable, unrelenting neck or upper extremity pain coming from the neck, would be to seek help at an urgent care clinic. Urgent care clinic wait times are slightly longer than most primary care physician offices on average. Again, it is important that one asks the question, "Am I seeking urgent pain control, or am I trying to determine what is causing the neck pain?"

While wait times around the primary care physician's office can typically be somewhere under an hour, it is important to understand that axial neck pain is not considered an emergency, and therefore it will not be given priority over patients deemed to have urgent conditions (eg. appendicitis).

Neck pain is only considered an emergency unless the pain is so severe, to such great extent, that the health care provider such

---

33 These clinics, which can include primary care office, neurosurgery and orthopedic spine clinics, and pain management clinics with 'extended' hours are region specific, and depends on availability, where an appointment is usually required. The most efficient way way to find out what is available is often to make a call.

as a triage nurse believes that it could have deterimental medical effects, such as to the cardiovascular system (breathing, elevated blood pressure, etc.) and/or some element of one's history indicates the need for more urgent work-up (see red flag symptoms), such as a fall with a suspected cervical spine fracture. This is not common, since pain of this severity occurs in conjunction with a trauma or neurologic deficit, both of which end up going to the emergency department for evaluation. Urgent care centers have a system of prioritizing the more urgent patients. This is a process known as triage. Regardless of the extent of pain, expect to receive a low priority and as a result the wait times are longer, varying from one hour to four hours, depending on how busy that facility is and the urgency level of other patients that are being seen.

Population Growth And Alternative Healthcare Options

The driving force behind the growth in healthcare options stems from population growth and how certain resources are overutilized. For example, The National Hospital Ambulatory Medical Care Survey estimates that up to half of all ER visits are for non-urgent care, which is defined by the American College of Emergency Physicians observation that 92% of emergency visits are patients needed care within minutes to approximately 2 hours.[34] In the past several decades, the growth in number of physicians trained, available hospital beds, emergency room capacity, and other facilities needed to care for people urgently (ie. for neck pain), has been outpaced by the

34 *https://www.debt.org/medical/emergency-room-urgent-care-costs/ accessed July 1, 2020.*

demand. As a result, episodes of low back and neck pain that are initially evaluated in an urgent setting end up being triaged and referred to an outpatient clinic setting, which in some regions leads to an appointment several weeks later. There are three very common (traditional) locations for back and neck pain to be evaluated, and that includes an urgent care clinic (acute care clinic), the hospital emergency department, and a primary care office (outpatient clinic).

Emergency Department

As mentioned above, neck pain symptoms alone, as well as low back pain receives relatively lower priority in the emergency department (ED). Historically, wait times for patients with these symptoms and no other red flag symptoms or concerning history can be a very time consuming process. An otherwise healthy person is commonly assigned a low priority in the emergency department. It is also the most expensive of the locations we discussed to get similar treatments. This is apart from anomalous services arising in the last decade such as the concierge healthcare model.[35] Neck and acute low back pain without 'red flag conditions', if at all possible.

Triaging Neck Pain

35 *Concierge services provide 24/7 primary care physician access, at a premium. Most often, this provides continuity of care, at all times, with a physician that is familiar with his/her medical history, giving one the ability to connect in a variety of methods such as text messaging or mobile phone for a flat-rate monthly fee plus charges per each specific service. This is becoming increasingly more common. (source: https://www.consumerreports.org/healthcare-costs/concierge-medical-care-pros-and-cons/ September 12, 2018)*

Overall, the ED which typically serves an entire region, was not designed to handle routine back and neck pain, which typically fills dozens of waiting rooms in most primary clinics. After all, this is the most common reason for an adult to go to the primary care office. On the other end of the spectrum, trauma is one instance where an emergency department is the most reasonable setting for an evaluation. For the most part, unless you are unable to carry out basic daily activities such as walking and self-care (eg. eating and getting dressed), an urgent care clinic, primary care clinic, or other specialist clinic would be a more appropriate setting for seeking initial care.

Nursing triage is a common process for ambulatory patients, on arrival at the ED, to assess the urgency of patient's needs. Due to the relatively low urgency assigned to neck pain, this drives up wait times for patients seeking acute back and neck pain care.

Many hospitals, internationally as well, in looking to improve this metric, have employed primary care services within the ED to primary care staff. In this system, triage can include placing patients on the path to being seen by general practicioners and emergency nurse practicioners within the hospital.[36]

ED Wait Times

The time it takes to be seen by a healthcare provider after entering the ED is the longest of the three options, and this is because patients with life-threatening and other urgent conditions are steadily entering the ED and being prioritized for care (triage). Basically, in an emergency department, uncomplicated neck pain work up will go at a slow place, as the process of diagnosis and

---

36 *Goncalves-Bradley D et al. Primary care professionals providing non-urgent care in hospital emergency departments. Cochrane Database Syst Rev. 2(2):2018*

treatment will have a low priority.

The ED Is The Most Expensive Venue For Neck and Back Pain Care

Urgency comes at a high price, which is rising at an incredible rate of 176% in the past decade, according to the nonprofit Health Care Cost Institute (HCCI).[37] Claims data from UnitedHealth Group shows the average cost of of 'avoidable' medical problems such as acute neck pain to be twelve times that of the cost in a physician's office.[38] Beyond this, numerous dynamics at play in the ED and many historical, social, and economic factors make the ED the worst option for most episodes of acute neck and LBP.

Another consideration with entering the ED is that the cost of care is much higher than if you were to get the treatment in the urgent care or primary care clinic.

Urgent Care Clinic

Urgent care clinics, defined as still a 'walk-in' clinic, arose out of a need for cost-effective and efficient care options for common painful conditions. As mentioned above, average ED costs dwarf those in the primary care clinic by an average of 12 times in the HCCI study. In another study, freestanding and hospital-based EDs were compared to urgent care centers in 16 metropolitan regions of Texas totalling 84% of the state population, and using

---

37 *Altucker K. USA Today: 'Really Astonishing': Average cost of hospital ER visit surges 176% in a decade, report says. June 4, 2019. https://www.usatoday.com/story/news/health/2019/06/04/hospital-billing-code-changes-help-explain-176-surge-er-costs/1336321001/*

38 *The High Cost of Avoidable Hospital Emergency Department Visits, accessed July 22, 2019. https://www.unitedhealthgroup.com/newsroom/posts/2019-07-22-high-cost-emergency-department-visits.html*

healthcare insurance data to assess relative cost. In the study, in 2015, average freestanding and hospital-based ED visit costs were $2,199 and $2,259, respectively, and only $168 at urgent care centers![39] Hospital-based urgent care clinics are excellent for painful neck and low back pain requiring same-day attention. Examples of conditions commonly requiring urgent attention (as typically advertised on websites from various urgent care clinics) include: a cut that may require stitches, but does not have significant bleeding, and also sprains, strains, and back and neck pain.

Primary Care Clinic

As mentioned in several other areas of this handbook, primary care clinics handle the most common patient complaint next to the common cold- which is low back pain. The physicians and providers in the primary care clinic are experts at appopriate evidenced-based treatment. This means that one is less likely to end up with second and third-line treatments and advanced imaging upfront. This includes cervical and lumbar MRIs, injections, and controlled substance prescriptions. Recalling the 2017 American College of Physicians Guidelines, the goal is to avoid as much treatment as possible in the first three months, since acute neck pain typically subsides within three months.

Another advantage of the primary care clinic is that preauthorization is more likely to be obtained for imaging studies, referrals, and advanced tests and treatments. Some insurance companies are denying coverage of these expensive and invasive diagnostic tests in the first three months. Keep this in mind, that if one goes to the ED and an MRI is recommended, insurance may not cover it.

---

39 *Ho V et al. Comparing Utilization and Costs of Care in Freestanding Emergency Departments, Hospital Emergency Departments, and Urgent Care Centers. Ann Emerg Med. 70(6):846-857:2017.*

One last point to keep in mind with primary care clinics is that you have the chance to obtain care for a problem that will more than likely require follow-up for, and unlike in an urgent or emergent setting, in the clinic you have the opportunity to go over your treatment options with a physcian or provider who you have developed a relationship with.

12 What Are The Roles of The Pain Management Doctor?

Pain management offices are outpatient clinics consisting of a physician-led multidisciplinary team with the common goal of improving quality of life and functional indepence by treating and curing pain. These specialists very often require a referral. Referrals allow the primary care physician to determine the medical necessity of seeing a specialist and also to limit the wait times by increasing access by those deemed appropriate for the referral. One example would be that a patient sees their family provider for angina, and after a workup, a small portion may require a cardioloist, cardiothoracic surgeon, and maybe even a gastroenterologist for reflux that presented as sternal discomfort. Interestingly, some clinics due not require a referral. Then, one has to confirm that their own insurance policy does not require a referral.

One common pattern arising are direct referrals to 'spine specialists'. Due to the very high volume of acute onset low back pain, and the complexity involved in the general work-up, and the existence of potential medico legal issues of the nature of the disease problems, patients are being referred directly to specialists for acute workup for generalized back and neck treatment.

Meanwhile, American Family Physician Society guidelines specify which types of imaging and acute pain treatments are acceptable in the first 3 months of pain, due to limitations in physician access, it is commonplace that specialists such as neurosurgeons and various other providers assist in the care of an acute neck and low back pain patient.

Overall, out of the needs of society, various specialists assist with the care of the low back pain patient with the intention to decrease wait times. Most pain management offices evaluate patients after having been recommended for referral by your established primary care doctor or provider. These offices specialize in acute and chronic pain - offering the widest range of available treatment options for spinal pain. This office has the greatest expertise to tailor pain treatments to each individual.

Historically, chronic pain treatment included long term use of prescription medications, with a high likelihood that opiates were integral to that treatment. Due to the increase in opiate-related deaths, chronic opiate treatment is being avoided. **As a result of increased regulation regarding opiate prescriptions, the overall effect has been less prescribing of opiates, careful transition to non-opiate analgesic therapy, and increased referrals to pain management offices for the treatment and prescribing of medication for acute and chronic back pain.**

Pain Management Appointments and Other Considerations

A pain management office is an outpatient (ambulatory) clinic setting that requires a referral prior to the appointment. Typically, the wait times are growing as a result of the aforementioned changes. **While some clinics allow same day scheduling, it is advisable to inquire prior to arriving for an unsched-**

uled visit. Multiple visits may often be required as well. One should develop a relationship with the provider that he or she is most comfortable with. Again, it is prudent to call and discuss what therapies are offered before scheduling and waiting for an appointment. Some offices do not offer certain interventional procedures and some offices have restrictions regarding pain management.

What does one do if they are in terrible pain, and all of these clinics are unavailable?

If one is unable to carry out basic functions in a reasonable time, and other self-care activities, a trip to the emergency department or urgent care clinic may be warranted. At these locations, one can get triaged promptly to be seen. While acute pain can be treated, the approach will be similar to the American College of Physicians 2017 guidelines.

Common Pain Management Services

- Aid in the diagnosis and treatment of chronic neck and arm pain: which can be difficult to distinguish from regional joint pathogy and other serious underlying conditions.
- Prescribe FDA-approved medications and other evidenced-based therapies (supported by research studies) that relieve

acute and chronic pain in line with evidenced-based guidelines. Abiding by the aforementioned guidelines is important in an era where there are numerous novel treatments that either lack high quality clinical studies to support their use, or lack any kind of long term follow-up.

- Provide diagnostic injections with the intent of identifying a pain generator, such as the shoulder, or cervical facet joint in the spine. Diagnostic injections are helpful because often they allow for both diagnosis and treatment of the cause of pain.

- Some pain management physicians provide advanced treatments, such as spinal cord stimulator placement, one possible treatment for certain types of back and neck pain (see section, spinal cord stimulation).

Legislation And Opiate Guidelines

Due to legislation in opiate prescribing practices, many healthcare institutions have outlined strict guidelines for the prescribing of opiates. In fact, most guidelines mirror the state-specific guidelines (see below for one example).[40] One of the most common guidelines the author has observed, is for practices to curtail the use of opiates outside of cancer pain; ie. to greatly limit prescribing of opiates for spinal degenerative diseases (prescriptions of controlled substances for greater than 3 months). The end result of this complexity and constant change in regulation has been for most providers to cease with chronic pain management for patients and to refer them to a pain management practice. This is especially the

40 *Opioid Prescribing Guidelines, State of Pennsylvania, one highlighted example, accessed August 1, 2020; https://www.health.pa.gov/topics/disease/Opioids/Pages/Prescribing-Guidelines.aspx*

case when opiates are potentially needed for chronic pain. One common exception to this rule, as mentioned has been with patients with terminal or cancer-related pain. This group of patients have been excluded from most of the recent guidelines. Overall, this is a relatively small population of patients.

Pain Management Specialties

The pain management physician and his/her team specializes in the short and long term treatment of pain, offering a comprehensive diagnostic and treatment program for a particular problem. Most pain management physicians are fellowship-trained pain specialists. This list is expanding and there are now at least six specialties whose boards allow their diplomates to be certified in pain medicine.

Understanding A Physician or Provider's Philosophy of Pain Management

Understanding a physician's overall pain management philosophy is important— This is especially relevant in spinal pain management. With chronic neck pain, a long term doctor-patient relationship will be established. This long term relationship should be established with likeminded goals as the patient. This provider should be interested in discussing these goals— their aim is to help their patients achieve success.

One example to illustrate this point would be a patient that had a history of a family member with opiate addiction. They are very anxious because they are afraid of becoming addicted as well. They do not want to be in a position where they are encouraged to take opiates— and with the chronic pain this patient is having, they are not entirely confident they will be able to decline any chance to obtain relief. Other patients are often placed in the position that they cannot be prescribed medications due to their occupation, such is the case of a school bus driver or police officer. In summary, one should have expectations that their treatment plan should be in line with your needs, which incorporates ones goals and values.

The Initial Pain Management Appointment

Often, an initial evaluation may not be with a pain management doctor, but rather with another practicioner (nurse practitioner or physician assistant) on the team. These team members are closely supervised and carefully trained by the pain manangement physician. The physician is responsible for all of the recommendations that their team members are providing. Since there are so many people with back and neck pain seeking care by a pain management doctor, this arrangement allows for one to be seen in a reasonable amount of time.

Pain Management Clinics Offer much More options Than Prescriptions

Concerns about pain management clinics stem from the negative attention that they have received due to the most recent opiate epidemic. This fear stems from the misconception that these clinics primarily treat pain with opiate prescriptions. One misconception would be to equate methadone clinics to pain clinics. Baby boomers witnessed the rise of methadone and the methadone clinic as a means of treatment for heroin and narcotic addiction as early as the 1970s. The prevailing image of these clinics in US culture was thought to be with the representation in one popular film movie titled *Trash*, which was produced by Andy Warhol in 1970. [41] And ever since the post- Vietnam era to the present, for 50 years, this has been a prevailing image of opiates and pain management in the US population. In actuality, opiate treatment for pain (eg. hydrocodone, oxycodone, etc.) represents a very small component of spinal pain management because they are ineffective, and have a high addiction potential and other side effects.

Pain management doctors are an appropriate referral for initial nonsurgical care of a patient with a degenerative spinal disorder, due to the wider range of appropriate therapies that they can provide from their office. Whereas, in a surgeon's clinic, the main tool of treatment is surgery, which is only needed by a fraction of patients. Often, some clinics are organized so that pain management doctors will establish a treatment plan, and for patients that end up needing surgery, they see the surgeon who is part of the same multispecialty clinic.

Commonly, for severe and disabling pain not alleviated by medications, a pain management physician can provide injections of medication into the spine, which are guided by x-rays and delivered precisely aroujnd the inflammed nerve. This provides higher concentrations of steroids, anti-inflammatory medication, or analgesic medication to the area that is needed- which explains why an injection can be so much more helpful for patients than oral medications.

Oral medications are less potent because they can be distrib-

41 *Hooked: Drug War Films In Britain, Canada, and the U.S. by Susan Boyd, 2007.*

uted throughout the body, potentially causing more negative side-effects. These injections a versatile, and in addition to injections around the nerve, they can be injected into numerous joint capsules at a site of suspected pain, and superficially into the muscles. The degree of pain relief may be helpful in patients with suspected pain coming from multiple sources, as it helps physicians understand all of the causes of pain in a particular person. Many pain management physicians provide a number of other targeted treatments, called interventional pain treatments, which will be discussed in the upcoming section on non-surgical treatments.

Summary

Overall, pain management facilities are very useful resources for aiding in the diagnostic workup and therapeutic care of chronic spinal pain. They are being utilized extensively in the community, in part due to their expertise in medical pain management as well as in the the safe and up to date recommendations for the prescription of analgesics. As a result, historically, the wait times to obtain these appointments have been increasing. In order to obtain the most efficient use of your first visit, set expectations, ask questions in advance, and come prepared.

13 **Muscle Strain and Physical Therapy**

The majority of acute and chronic neck pain cases can be attributed to the muscles of the neck, or inflammation within the muscles and the overlying connective tissue. A 'pulled muscle', describes muscle that is overused, overstretched, or torn, resulting in inflammation in the muscle. This is also referred to as a **muscle strain**. This is the most common cause of neck pain, and it is much more common than a spinal degenerative problem. This should not come as a suprise, as this problem occurs with great frequency in all of the other orthopedic joints. Muscle strain becomes especially troublesome in the neck, as the the musculature is extensive (Fig 13-1) and vital for a greater range of motion and freedom.

Muscle Strain In The Neck

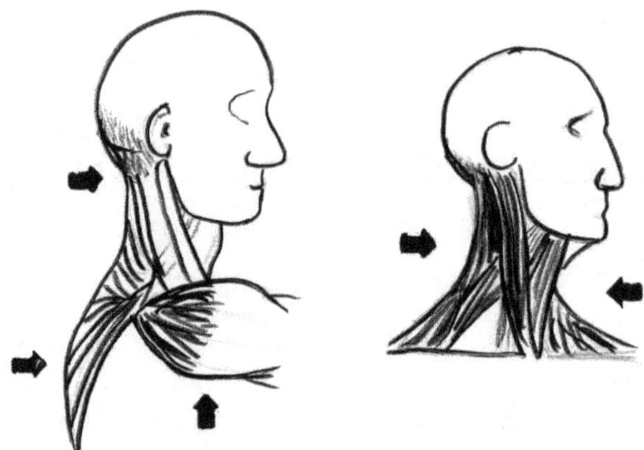

Figure 13-1. The Neck is among the most complex regions of the body in terms of compound movements and function (view, left image; anterior view with maximal neck rotation, right image). These muscles (arrows) allow for rotation, flexion, extension, lateral bending, and translation. Muscle strain can involve any muscle groups inserting in the thoracic spine, scapula, clavicle, humerus, occiput, and sternum.

First, How is Muscle Strain Diagnosed?

Muscle strain is an unpopular diagnosis because there is no definitive imaging test that can diagnose muscle strain. One obstacle to using MRI (the penultimate tool for diagnosis) to diagnose muscle strain is the large number of layered, small muscle groups with layers of muscle that weave in and out of the images. Second, routine muscle strain does not produce unique neck muscle characteristics. The next obstacle with MRI is that with high probability, numerous degenerative spinal disease manifestations will be find on any MRI. Therefore, in almost all cases of muscle strain, the use of a cervical MRI will result in the clinician identifying degenerative spinal findings and not muscle strain.

Ultimately, just by a description of the clinical history should be adequate, without a cervical MRI. Typically a clinical history of muscle stain would include some event involving overuse of neck muscles, significant neck discomfort with neck motion, and the absence of other concerning findings, such as numbness, weakness, and pain travelling down the extremity. Also, the pain should improve over a period of days to weeks, improve with over-the-counter anti-inflammatory medication, heat, ice, massage, rest, and avoiding strenuous activity.

Overuse is a Hallmark of Muscle Strain

A muscle strain is brought on by overexertion, as well as heavy and repetitive movements. Often, the muscle strain can peak the following 1-2 days after overuse. The pain does not travel away from the neck, and is not associated with numbness or weakness. Some patients describe muscular strain as something they woke up with. This pain is made much worse with any kind of neck movement, since it is the inflammation of the neck muscles that is the primary cause of the problem. The natural course of inflammation, will be gradual improvement without any intervention. MRI is a poor tool (or any other imaging) to diagnose paraspinal muscle strain and cannot be made with imaging of any kind, including an MRI. However, in some specialty academic centers, use of the 'muscle function' MRI study has been an ongoing investigational persuit for more than ten years. In this author's opinion, it is only a matter of time before one of the most common symptoms gets itself a definitive diagnostic test to correlate muscle injury to neck strain.[42]

Paraspinal muscles generally refer to muscle groups adjacent to

---

42 *Cagnie B et al. Use of muscle functional magnetic resonance imaging to compare cervical flexor activity between patients with whiplash-associated disorders and people who are healthy. Phys Ther. 90(8):1157-64, 2010.*
Cagnie B et al. Functional reorganization of cervical flexor activity because of induced muscle pain evaluated by muscle functional magnetic resonance imaging. Man ther. 16(6):470-5, 2011.

the spine). A muscle is strained, and the term sprain is a separate problem and more commonly is used to describe a stretch or ligament tear. Ligaments connect bone to other bone, and require much greater forces to injure, and are much more serious. More recent ligamentous injuries can often be seen on an MRI.

What Can I Do if I Have a Muscle Strain?

Again, it can not be overstated that an MRI does not clearly diagnose the most common cause of neck pain, which is the paraspinal muscle strain. Also, as mentioned above, odds are that an MRI will identify spinal degeneration and potentially lead to the persuit additional workup and treatment. Again, MRI will not diagnose muscle strain. For this reason (and others), it has been more common for some time to see insurance companies and other payers to put barriers in place to early (in the first 3 months) cervical MRI acquisition for acute neck pain in the first three months.[43] Instead, physical therapy is becoming a more common recommendation prior to obtaining an MRI.

Poor Neck Posture: Affect and Effect

---

43 *MRI very clearly shows normal aging of the spine and related processes such as cervical degenerative disc disease and spondylosis. This is often a red herring and statistically less likely to be causing neck pain. This is because of the numerous interdigitated pattern of muscles arrange from very short muscles that are deep and attached along the spine to some of the larger muscle groups in your body such as your latissimus dorsi, rhomboids, and trapezius muscles.*

Neck posture can be a manifestation both a manifestation of a neck problem as well as a cause of neck pain. Both forward head and protracted shoulder posture are two involuntary postures that are thought to contrinbute to the development of chronic neck pain (Fig 13-2).[44]

Forward Head and Protracted Shoulder Posture Can Contribute To Neck Pain

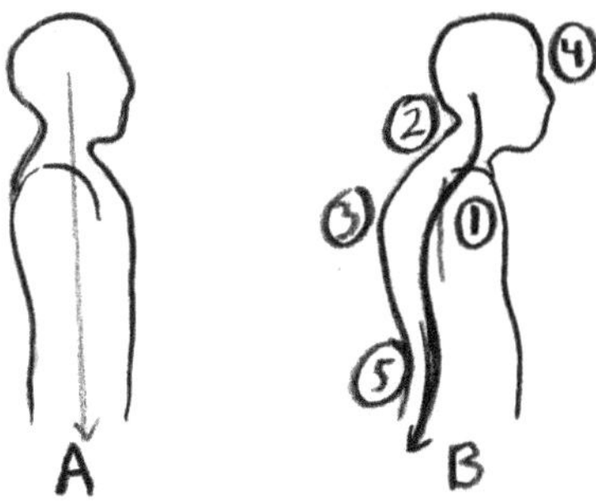

Figure 13-2. Chronic voluntary postural deviations can contribute to chronic neck pain. In the normal posture (A), the head, neck, shoulders, and spine form a straight line. 'Protracted shoulders' describes that characteristic forward position of the shoulders seen most often in adolescence (1). Other compensations that are typically seen in association include a forward head position (4), exaggerated cervical extension to maintain a horizontal line of sight (2), as well as spinal compensations in the thoracic(3) and lumbar spine (5) to balance the head over the pelvis.

Years of postural habit can be hard to overcome. It is thought that most of this postural habit is more of a consequence of ergonomics and increasingly more common in adolescence due to the

---

44 *Diepenmaat CM et al. Neck/shoulder, low back, and arm pain in relation to computer use, physical activity, stress, and depression among Dutch adolescents. Pediatrics. 117:412-416, 2006.*

increased prevalence of smartphone and other portable digital device use as well as computers in the present generation of adolescents.[45] Recognition of this possible hazard due to increased use of these technologies can be helpful to help improve quality of life, at the cost of voluntary awareness of the problem and consistency.[46]

Poor posture resembles a forward-leaning position of the shoulders and upper arms, which can either result in an exaggerated extension of the neck and anterior position of the head. When the head is anterior to the spine, muscles will be under a state of increased tension and in a state of maximum length. In general, deviations from normal spinal alignment lead to increased pain, a pattern identified long ago by spinal deformity and scoliosis experts.

Abnormal Neck Posture As A Manifestation of Muscle Spasm or Nerve Compression

Generally, preventable causes of neck pain are encountered in younger patients, whereas in older patients abnormal neck postures are often a manifestation of an underlying problem such as a degenerative condition of the spine, or nerve compression. In general, abnormal neck postures are observed in severe stenosis that causes painful nerve compression. For example, if a nerve is compressed as it exits (in the neural foramen) the left side of the spine, it is common to see a patient bending their head to the right, as this tends to open the left neural foramen to a slight degree and decrease pain. Similarly, patients with central canal stenosis tend to flex their head forward- often this decreases central canal stenosis.

---

45 *van Niekerk et al. Photographic measurement of upper-body sitting posture of high school students: a reliability and validity study. BMC Musculoskelet Disord. 9:113, 2008.*

46 *Ruivo RM, et al. Effects of a Resistance and Stretching Training Program on Forward Head and Protracted Shoulder Posture In Adolescents. J Manip and Phys Ther. 1(40):1-10, 2017*

Ergonomics At Work

An ergonomic position refers to a body's alignment that is both held still for a prolonged time period (static position) and at the same time closely resembles the normal anatomic body alignment. Ergonomic positions are only achieved due to awareness. One example is used in the illustration below. Notice that the patient is bringing his whole body to the horizontal line of sight with the monitor (Fig. 13-3). In order to do this correctly, the monitor, chair, and table should instead be brought into a horizontal line of sight with the employee, while keeping the spine neutral (Fig. 13-4).

Computer monitor, chair, desk, and keyboard adjustments are essentail to keeping a proper ergonomic alignment in order to avoid both chronic neck and low back pain both at home and at the workplace. Most people that develop ergonomic related neck pain spend a significant amount of time positioned improperly while at a desk, using a monitor, hand-held phone, driving a vehicle, or using machinery. Being attentive to one's ergonomics and these common scenarios can help avoid workplace eregonomics becoming a contributor to chronic neck pain. For additional questions about workplace ergonomics, please refer to the question in the following section about various workplace-related changes that can be made to avoid neck pain.

Adjust The Computer Display (And Not The Neck) To

Meet Your Line of Sight

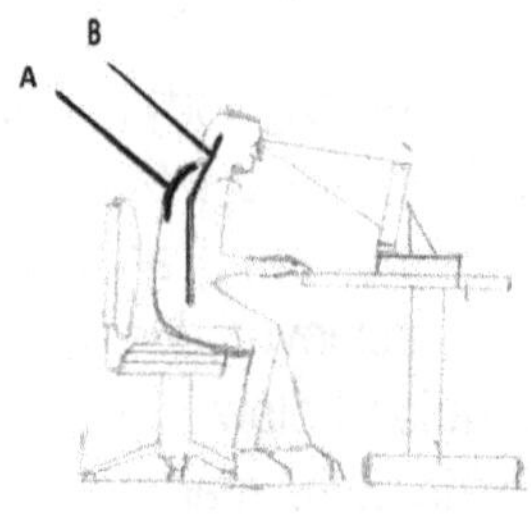

Figure 13-3. Poor Ergnomics. A monitor positioned too low causes painful spine (A) and neck flexion (B).

Proper Ergonomics: Keeping a Neutral Spinal Alignment At The Work Station

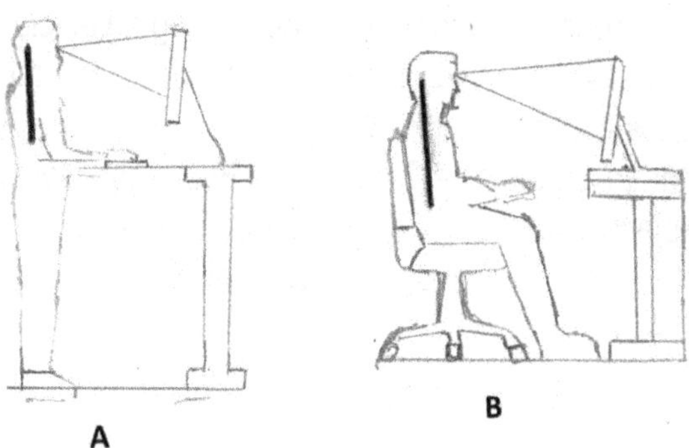

Figure 13-4. Notice that regardless of using a standing desk(A) or sitting in a traditional work setting (B), a neutral spinal alignment (vertical dark line) is seenin both cases. A neutral spinal alignment is only possible when your monitor is in your horizontal line of sight.

Even a mild injury can cause soft tissue and muscle injury. This can range from mild overexertion with physical activity, a sports-related collision during a recreational activity or severe injury from a motor-vehicle collision. Regardless of the mechanism, with trauma, see a professional to help make sure potentially serious injuries are identified early. Regarding soft tissue injury, healing is slow, and even slower the older one gets.

Even mild injury to the muscles and soft tissue in the neck (and low back) can take months to properly heal and for pain to significantly improve. It is important that for minor sports or fitness-related injuries to reduce physical activity, allowing proper time for recovery. Complete removal from physical activity altogether is not advised.

Again, be cognizant of red flag symptoms and consult a physician early when appropriate (see red flag chapter with any questions regarding warning signs and symptoms). For the most part, outside of trauma, there are no surgical treatments for painful soft tissue injuries of the spine *per se*. Again, soft tissue injury is very difficult to properly diagnose with an MRI. As a result, degenerative spinal problems are usually implicated when an MRI is obtained. This can often lead you down the wrong path to treatment.

Neck Pain

The best initial treatment for uncomplicated neck pain is daily and consistent stretching, core strengthening, and other conditioning exercises. This is the least invasive treatment for acute neck pain and arguably should be utilized more than it currently is. Often, over-the-counter analgesics are helpful to provide enough pain relief to over come the initial pain of starting a physical therapy regimen. It is seldomly recommended to avoid any activity during the acute pain period. However, it would be advisable to avoid heavy and strenuous activity, which it is particularly the kind of activity that could've caused the onset of neck pain.

Physical therapists and their staff help with core strengthening, which is a great way to improve posture, and improve overall quality of life. In some studies, patients with acute neck pain who were referred to physical therapy for 8-12 weeks were less likely to require advanced spinal imaging or further testing. One rationale for this protocol and a partial explanation why this protocol works is that it required patients to wait 3 months. As we have discussed, most acute episodes of neck pain will go away without intervention during 3 months. Overall, physical pherapy is a good initial therapy for acute neck pain, even if it doesn't take immediate effect as with medications. This is because of how safe it is. It carries a fraction of the risks that have been reported with some other therapies.

Physical Therapists Specializing in Spinal Conditions?

For the most part, there are self-designated spine subspecialists among the physical therapy centers. However, it is rare to find physical therapists exclusively seeing spinal patients and determining the capabilities of your local physical therapy clinic is fairly easy. Physical therapists trained in 'mechanical diagnosis and therapy' or the McKenzie Method (M.D.T.) can be helpful, which is a spine speciality certification in physical therapy. Is MDT essential to obtaining physical therapy? One recent 2020 study reviewing the literature on neck pain found insufficient evidence that patients managed by MDT had significant improvements in pain or function.[47] Nonetheless, many patients find this to be of particular benefit; this process works towards localizing pain caused by most musculoskeletal problems. Overall, most physical therapists can provide safe and helpful care for You.

The Initial Appointment

The inital appointment is much like a doctor's initial care visit, where over the course of approximately 45 minutes you will meet with a physical therapist. The physical therapist helps coordinate and develop a treatment plan during this initial assessment. This includes discussing medical problems, pain, functioning, and assessing overall medical wellness. After this is done, a working diagnosis is made, and a treatment plan with goals are created. This plan outlines all the treatments that you need, how often you will need them, and how long your course of therapy will be. There may or may not be a follow-up appointment to reassess your pro-

---

47 *Edmond SL et al. Cognitive Behavioural Interventions, and Function and Pain Outcomes Among Patients With Chronic Neck Pain Managed With The McKenzie Approach. Musculskeletal Care. 18(10):46-52*

gress. In some practices, your time spent with a physical therapist will be limited, due to the high demand. You will be more than likely spending your time with a physical therapy assistant (PTA), who will guide you through each step of your session. The PTA will help you go through the prescribed treatments appropriately, and safely. This is important for the spine to prevent injury.

14 What Can a Chiropractor Do For Me?

One answer might be that a chiropractor provides spinal manipulation and other manual treatments such as adjustments and traction to relieve pressure on the nerve roots, thus healing neck and low back pain. However, spinal manipulation therapy (SMT) or chiropractic, is another term for treatment provided by chiropractors who contend that this alternative medical therapy lends itself to correct a whole host of medical problems, including non-orthopedic issues, through the restoration of normal spinal alignment. In, *Chiropractic: The Superior Alternative*, the author, William Koch, became interested and entered the field of chiropractic when he realized that his childhood medical ailments were finally cured when he went to see a chiropractor. In it, he states, "I am still very susceptible to bronchial, sinus, and throat infections, unless I am able to keep my spine in good adjustment. When I am in adjustment, I do great."[48]

---

48 *Chiropractic: The Superior Alternative, by William Koch, p. 11.*

Since its inception with the first case report of spinal adjustment as an ad hoc treatment for heart disease by D.D. Palmer in 1906, the field of chiropractic asserts a synchronistic relationship between spinal alignment and the immune system.[49] It may be defined as manual therapy, mobilization, and/or maneuvers ('adjustments') that have the goal of relieving spinal nerve compression and ultimately relieving sciatica and/or neck and low back pain. Overall, SMT and other forms of 'alternative medicine' therapies are growing, as observed in a five-year study of the national health interview survey conducted by a division of the CDC (Fig. 14-1).

Increased Use of Chiropractic and Other Alternative Medicine Therapies For Acute Pain In The Past 12 Months, 2012 vs 2017, National Health Interview Survey

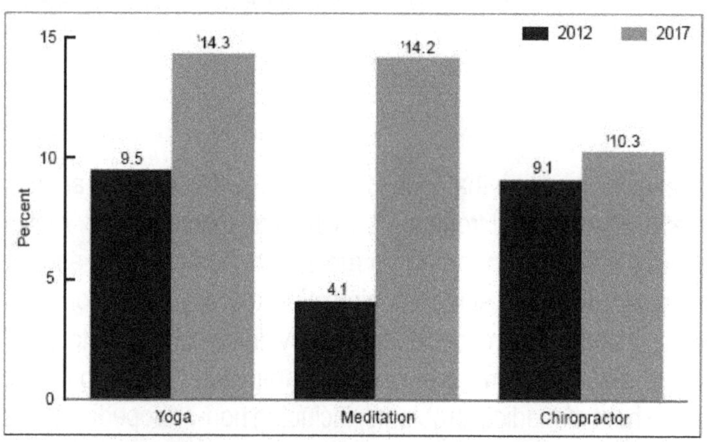

Figure 14-1. 5 year interim analysis of alternative medicine treatments for acute pain over a 12 month period, showing the overall growth of yoga, meditation, and chiropractic. Source: National Health Interview Survey[50]

---

49 *In, The Science of Chiropractic; its principles and adjustments, 1st ed. Daniel David Palmer and Bartlett Joshua Palmer, Davenport. IA: Palmer School of Chiropractic, 1906. https://library.palmer.edu/greenbooks/Vol 1.*

50 *https://www.cdc.gov/nchs/data/databriefs/db325-h.pdf*

PT and SMT Evidence Using Meta-analysis and Systematic Review

The mechanism of how physical therapy and SMT alleviates pain from a disc herniation is least understood by patients. If this is a tough concept to grasp, that is certainly okay, as it is the least understood concept by experts as well! Several studies have attempted to summarize the effects of SMT and to determine how well it reduces pain. Generally, a meta-analysis or systematic review are types of studies that attempt to answer a narrow research question using the available published research. This is a controversial process, as it is arguably impossible to add two completely different studies. High quality research is very costly to conduct, and in many instances, dozens of low-quality research studies are available that many tangentially address a topic. An attempt to 'normalize' these studies, a process to assign relative values to each study, so that the studies can be aggregated, is a highly controversial process. Opponents to this method argue that studies with very different designs can not be aggregated appropriately in a 'scientific' manner. However, since the majority of studies in many surgical specialties are of a lower cost and lower quality design, there is certainly a benefit to conducting a systematic review of the published literature. In the author's opinion, the benefit comes from being able to read a short systematic review and gain the benefit of insight while simultaneously avoiding the chore of reading a thousand pages of the individual studies. This is not feasible to do for every medical topic- reviews in general are helpful.

Another point is inescapable, which is that low-quality studies are limited in terms of the strength of the conclusions that can be made, whether it be 1 study versus 100 studies. However, many agree that there is tremendous value from analyzing the results of 10,000 patients across studies of mixed quality, especially if there are concordant findings. In summary, keep in mind that a systematic review is not the final word on a subject.[51]

Physical Therapy and Spinal Manipulation Therapy: Appropriate Treatments For Uncomplicated Acute Neck Pain

Physical therapy(PT) and spinal manipulation(chiropractic) are two common recommendations that patients encounter at the onset of acute neck pain. Interestingly, this widespread enrollment of patients or self-referral to either PT and/or SMT occurs despite there being a clear explanation as to how this treatment works. In 2017, one literature review by Fredin and Loras compared the treatment effects of either SMT or PT, or both SMT and PT in combination. Their study attempted to review the literature and to compary and summarize the treatment effects of the three groups. They set out to determine which of the aforementioned treatments were the most effective at reducing resting neck pain intensity, reducing overall disability due to neck pain, and the impact of these treatments on quality of life, which was analyzed immediately post-treatment, 6 months, and 1 year later. **They found 7 studies of moderate-quality, and ultimately concluded that there was no significant difference with either SMT, PT, or both SMT and PT combined in terms of reducing pain, disability and improving quality of life at any of the analyzed time points.**[52] It should be

51 *Gopalakrishnan S et al. Systematic reviews and meta-analysis: Understanding the best evidence in primary healthcare. J Family Med Prim Care. 2(1):9-14.*

52 *Fredin K and Loras H. Manual Therapy, exercise therapy or combined treatment in the management of adult neck pain - A systematic review and meta-analysis. Musculoskelet Sci Pract. 10(31):62-71:2017.*

noted that there was an improvement in pain, and therefore from this, either one of the preferred treatment options are acceptable at the onset of acute neck pain.

This is not the only review of the literature. In 2010, Miller and colleagues published a systematic review which found 17 randomized studies addressing this same question of effectiveness of SMT and PT. They found that combining SMT and PT led to a superior reduction in pain that exceeded either SMT or PT alone, but at the longest follow-up interim, there was no significant difference in effectiveness.[53] In other words, if no personal preference exists, a patient can have a discussion with a trusted spinal expert or healthcare provider and discuss with him or her what they suggest, since there is no clear answer. It should be noted, that while a clear mechanism for how these treatments is lacking, studies observe an improvement. **Unfortunately, in the setting of medical conditions like muscle strain and degenerative spinal conditions, spontaneous improvement (without any treatment) is the natural order of things. It is challenging both to design studies to enroll patients intended to find a clear and convincing treatment effect where a large number of patients begin to spontaneously improve without treatment.**

The Treatment Effectiveness of Spinal Manipulation: Further Hurdles

The question of the effectiveness of spinal manipulation has been periodically evaluated. There are plenty of literature reports of pain reduction with the use of manipulation, and it is also not hard to find an assessment of this literature quality. Regarding this, consider the editorial published in the *Journal of Pain and Symptom Management* "...Unfortunately, here in the United States, the

---

53 *Miller J et al. Manual therapy and exercise for neck pain: a systematic review. Man Ther. 15(4):334-45, 2010.*

lack of scientific plausibility and evidence of safety and efficacy for chiropractic is no barrier to chiropractice practice. Each of the 50 states separately regulates the practice and each, in one form or another, incorporates traditional chiropractic philosophy. This allows a scope of chiropractic practice approaching that of an allopathic primary care physician and permits chiropracters to make claims that would otherwise be fraudulent (e.g., the detection and correction of subluxations as essential to human health)..."[54]

Many questions about spinal manipulation remain unanswered by research, which include the most fundamental such as how the treatment actually works, but the details such as the frequency of treatments needed, the overall duration, and the long term effects. These unanswered questions lead to a lack of consistency regarding advice from healthcare providers, such as the expected duration of benefit of pain reduction to expect from SMT, the odds it will work with one treatment, and questions of effectiveness. These are just a few unanswered questions, but they run the whole gamut of how little is understood.

However, for many reasons, SMT will continue to grow as a popular treatment for acute neck and back pain. Consider just some alternative treatments and workups, such as physical therapy, injections, advanced diagnostic imaging, and prescription medications; These alternatives are more expensive, have addiction potential in the case of many analgesics, and are more invasive, with respect to injections. The cost of healthcare in 2016 was 18% of gross domestic product, or about 3 trillion dollars. In one *JAMA* study, back and neck pain was determined to be the most expensive condition of the 154 that were analyzed.[55] After this is considered, it is no surprise that insurance company approve certain low

---

54 *Bellamy, J. Re: Chiropractice: A Critical Evaluation. J Pain Symptom Manage. 36(3):E4, 2008.*

Ernst E. Chiropractic: a critical evaluation. J Pain Symptom Manage. 35:544-562, 2008.

55 *Dieleman JL et al. US Health Care Spending by Payer and Health Condition, 1996-2016. JAMA. 323(9):863-884.*

cost alternative medicine treatments in the hopes to contain costs related to far more expensive treatment and workup such as medical imaging and invasive treatments.

What are some of the Unique Risks Reported With Spinal Manipulation Therapy of the Neck?

Overall, reported complications from spinal manipulation range between one in a million and one out every thousand patients. Many of these risks stem from pre-existing medical conditions, such as severe stenosis, which is not often known prior to encountering these complications. For a detailed examination of the various complications that can arise from spinal manipulation, Swait and Finch published a review in The Journal, *Chiropractic and Manual Therapies* in 2017.[56]

Vertebral Artery Injury and Neck Manipulation: The Ongoing Debate

One concerning risk that has been reported to occur in association with spinal manipulation of the neck is cervical vertebral artery injury and stroke, which is potentially deadly. The vertebral artery supplies oxygenated blood to the cervical spinal cord, and brainstem, include many other critical areas whereby even the smallest embolic strokes can permanently incapacitate any patient. The research is heavily contested regarding the true relationship between neck manipulation and arterial injury. One major reason is that the

---

56 *Swait G and Finch R What are the risks of manual teratment of the spine? A scoping review for clinicians. Chropr Man Therap. 25(37):2017.*

incidence is fairly low. Still, all patients should be aware of the potential risks of devastating stroke, or spinal cord injury. For many physicians at some point in practice, cervical vertebral artery injury and strokes has been observed to occur in association, often with stroke as well.[57] However, some chiropracters argue that there is not enough data to prove a cause and effect relationship. This might be true, as quality of the published research is limited and of low quality.

Published in one chiropracter journal, one review draws conclusions of the unfounded relationship merely by a selective commentary of various studies that helps the authors make the most efficient argument— In doing so, they conclude that there is little to the concern regarding a relationship between manual neck manipulation and cervical artery dissection and/or stroke. To summarize, this is more of an issue of 'guilty by association' and less so a cause-effect relationship.[58] Another review by researchers Paulus and Thaler is strikingly unusual, as the research title is organized similar to a news headline, which is designed to deliver the point one intends to make without having to read the article, "Does case misclassification threaten the validity of studies investigating the relationship between neck manipulation and vertebral artery dissection stroke? Yes."[59]

One research article is illustrative of the general difficulty with

---

57 *Albuquerque FC et al. Craniocervical arterial dissections as sequelae of chiropractic manipulation: patters of injury and management. Cassidy JD et al. Risk of vertebrobasilar stroke and chiropractic care: results of a population-based case-control and case-crossover study. Spine 33(4 Suppl):S176-83:2008.*

58 *Moser N et al, Effect of cervical manipulation on vertebral artery and cervical haemodynamics in patients wijth chronic neck pain: a crossover randomised controlled trial.*

59 *Paulus JK and Thaler DE. Does case misclassification threaten the validity of studies invesetigating the relationship between neck manipulation and vertebral artery dissection stroke? Yes" Chiropr Man Therap. 24:42, 2016.*

interpreting novel research studies and drawing conclusions from them in the context of clinical applicability. Moser and colleagues evaluate the hemodynamics of the two vertebral arteries at the time of spinal manipulation of the neck in an attempt to show in a different way that the risk is unfounded. Upon reading it most people would interpret this as it does cast some doubt on the association between cervical vertebral artery injury and or manual manipulation. However, this study deserves some attention, as it illustrates the difficulty in designing studies and the limitations on any conclusions that can be made from incredibly narrow studies. There are serious design limitations with this study. First, the study design has an incredible number of patients excluded— Of 916 patients, only 20 patients are included (which is approximately 2%). For the most part, in order for a study to assess treatment effectiveness, and provide useful data for clinicians, inclusion and exclusion criteria should be similar to current practice and the number of subjects excluded should be kept at a minimum. Limiting the number of excluded patients that potentially could've been enrolled, especially beyond the normal, limits the patient population, or narrows it down— to the elite 2% of enrolees. If the methodology of the study is so foreign to common clinic practice— and it likely is, because many aspects are conducted differently, a health care provider would not be able to use a particular treatment and expect a similar result— and this is because all of the other practices are different. Not many chiropractic offices can likely attest that only 2% of their neck pain patients meet the criteria to be offered spinal manipulation therapy for the neck. Many other methods were clear, and without very specific methodology, other clinics cannot compare practices of a study and conclude that they should expect similar outcomes. It is not clear if any findings on an MRI prior to spinal manipulation were the cause of exclusion, and it appears they were not. However, of 916 patients, it would be surprising if there were not instances where pathologies other than spondylotic/degenerative conditions were identified and the patients were referred to spinal surgeons for evaluation (eg. fractures and spinal tumors). With such a high number of exclusions (98%), it is difficult to truly say that there is no evidence of decreased brain perfusion with spinal manipulation. Only under the characteristics of the remaining 2% of patients that made it through the rigorous exclusion criteria were these 20 patients observed to not have hemodynamic changes.

And so, this study does not contribute to the 'growing body of evidence' of the safety of spinal manipulations of the neck— and that of course is because the study did not demonstrate whether it emulated the chiropractic practice and the conditions under which these cases of cervical dissection occurred. It also cannot simply attribute serious devastating complications as 'protopathic bias'or 'reverse causality'. In the context of spine patients, these two terms are used to essentially imply that the initial neck pain that brought the patient in for treatment was actually the presenting symptoms of cervical vertebral artery disease and dissection in itself. This is a very valid concern raised by many experienced researchers in the field of spinal pain— The incidence of diagnosed cervical arterial dissection and/or stroke is so low, that this theory that the presenting neck pain was due to arterial injury has not been refuted, and the subsequent treatment of cervical dissection with spinal manipulation may or may not exacerbate the pre-existing disease process can certainly lead to a misplaced cause-effect relationship in these very uncommon clinical events.[60] Once again, these studies lack an appropriate design.

In the end, how a study is designed dictates the usefullness by other clinicians and the strength of the conclusions that can be made. Overall, the Moser study of brain perfusion in the events surrounding spinal manipulation did not attempt to emulate any

---

60 *Haldeman S. Clinical perceptions of the risk of vertebral artery dissection after cervical manipulation: The effect of referral bias. Spine J. 2(5):334-42, 2002.*

model of current practice, and is therefore of little relevace.

Summary

Overall, there are unique risks reported to be in association with spinal manipulation of the neck— some of which are potentially life-threatening and should not be cast aside and given the severity, patients should be made aware. There is support lending credence to both sides of the debate regarding spinal manipulation as a risk for dissection and stroke. Although alternative medicine techniques lack clear mechanisms as to how a benefit is perceived, and potentially, many of these alternative medicine techniques take credit for a disease process that naturally heals itself, they can be of benefit in chronic neck pain as well. To date, there is low quality evidence, but evidence nonetheless, in support of spinal manipulation for neck pain, with fairly low risk of serious injury.

15 What are the Specialties That Perform Spinal Surgery? (The Orthopedic and Neurological Surgeons)

The majority of degenerative spinal conditions can be equally addressed by either an orthopedic surgeon or a neurosurgeon. Nearly all patients that require surgery due to an underlying spinal degenerative condition (disc herniations included) can equally be treated by either specialty. Some of the differences will be briefly explained, but none of these differences should impact your decision to see a particular physician. The physician that you ultimately decide to see should be someone that you feel comfortable with to help develop a care plan.[61]

Orthopedic Spinal Surgery

Today, the management of spinal disorders has become so complex that many surgeons undertake an additional year after residency where they complete a 'fellowship training' in spine surgery. This is an additional year of training after residency. Orthopedics is a versatile operative field and typically the orthopedic surgeons that practice spinal surgery are fellowship-trained.

Spinal surgery comprises a greater portion of neurosurgery resident education, and for the most part, most neurosurgeons consider themselves capable in the surgical care of routine spinal problems for adults. Neurosurgeons have fellowship training in spinal surgery as well. Overall, the choice to undergo surgical care with a neurosurgeon or orthopedic surgeon has not been shown in research studies to influence surgical outcome, regarding the most common spinal degenerative conditions.

---

61 *Since the author is a neurosurgeon, any answer provided will contain a potential bias. Even when the recommendations are neutral in any issue, being neither for nor against something, there is still conscious and unconscious bias that cannot be completely eliminated. For that reason, studies that go through greater attempts to limit bias are considered the most impactful. Studies can be blinded to the subject receiving the treatment with a placebo, and they can be blinded to the clinician conducting the study with the use of a third party. Clinical studies like these are expensive and very difficult to design. For that reason, most studies will not be double-blinded and randomized. Wherever possible, when considering an action based on gathered information, ask yourself if that information has the potential for bias (examples are abundant).*

Neurological Surgery

While the same care can be provided by either neurosurgeons or orthopedic spinal surgeons for degenerative conditions, some spinal problems involving the spinal cord, disorders of spinal fluid flow, or any intradural surgery (Fig. 15-1) for that matter, are treated only by a neurosurgeon, as the microsurgical tools and techniques are very similar to some of those microsurgical techniques utilized during their training and for the majority of cranial surgery.

Intradural Spinal Surgery

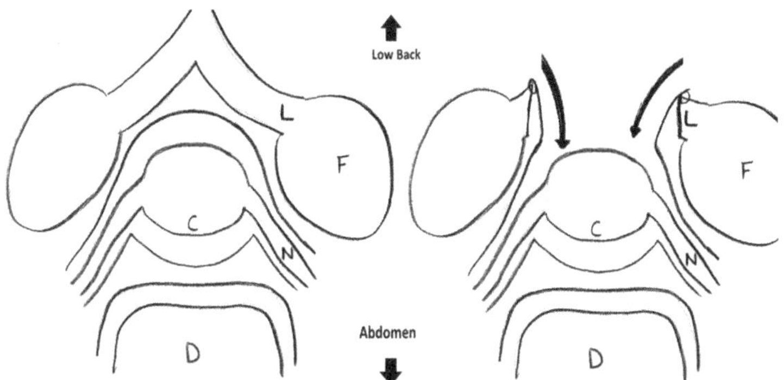

Figure 15-1. Intradural Surgery: The normal cross section of the spine is shown, where to the top of the image is the direction of the low back and the lower portion is in the direction of the abdomen (arrows). The spinal dura is a fibrous tissue layer that is continuous with the cranial dura that covers both the brain and spinal cord, and is filled with cerebrospinal fluid. The spinal cord (C) and nerve roots (N) are contained by the dura, and are normally (left image) protected anteriorly by the vertebral body and disc (D) and posteriorly by the lamina (L), on on the left and right-sides by the facets (F). The exiting nerves are in close proximity to the intervertebral disc (D).

Intradural surgery involves a posterior incision, a laminectomy, which is a surgical removal of the lamina, and temporary opening of the enveloping dura (right image). After opening the dura, it must be closed and be free of leaking under normal pressures. Almost all cranial surgery is intradural, and so the term intradural is not commonly used to describe cranial procedures. In comparison, most compressive spinal problems occur extradurally, or, outside of the dura, and therefore most surgery is extradural in the spine. For example, cervical intradural disc herniations are exceedingly rare,[62] and most disc herniations and stenosis occur outside of the dura.

The spinal cord has a leathery covering that holds in all of the cerebrospinal fluid, called the dura. For spinal diseases that require crossing this barrier, ie. opening the dura to operate on the spinal cord, a neurosurgeon typically handles this. Again, the overwhelming majority of spinal diseases are treated by either specialty, and each surgeon's unique training gives each and every surgeon a unique perspective. Moreover, AOSpine Europe, a European Academy of spinal surgery research and clinical care, issued a 60 question quiz to each of its 289 responding members (spinal surgeons), and they found no significant difference in the test knowledge between neurosurgeons and orthopedic surgeons with regard to the management of spinal surgery problems. While there are other studies that looked at this question, in general, there is no convincing argument that their is a difference in fund of knowledge between the two.

A Post-Residency Fellowship In Spinal Surgery

As research and innovation improves safety and patient outcomes in spinal surgery, certain diseases within the spinal surgery realm are particularly challenging. These historically include **sco-**

62 *Guan Q et al. Cervical intradural disc herniation: A systematic review. J Clin Neurosci. 48:1-6, 2018.*

liosis, pediatric spinal surgery where considerations have to be made in a spine that is growing, as well as spinal deformities where considerations have to be as to planning the correction or maintenance of the center of gravity. In any region of the spine, when there is rotation and deviation in the coronal plane (to the left or right of the body), scoliosis occurs (Fig. 15-2). When the head is too far pitched forward or backwards, it is referred to as sagittal plane deformity. Having a 'neutral global spinal alignment' refers to the head properly positoned over the pelvis, which in most people requires the least activation of spinal and lower extremity musculature and therefore limits daily energy expenature — This balance may be referred to as 'sagittal balance'.[63]

When the spine has a disease process effecting that balance, surgery may eventually become necessary. The treatment for global spinal malalignment in the adult (where the spine is no longer growing) is generally completed with a multilevel fusion using screws and rods and other corrective measures to return the spine to a normal alignment. These are complex lengthy procedures and is generally thought to be one area identified within spinal surgery that it may benefit the patient to seek care from a fellowship-trained surgeon.

A successful surgery does not stop at the door to the operating room, and the establishment of well-developed postoperative care programs with physical therapists and experienced nursing teams who are knowledge about scoliosis usually leads to the better outcomes. In terms of general knowledge base, surgeons that completed a one-year fellowship demonstrated on testing, a significantly greater knowledge base in the area of spinal deformity surgery compared to spinal surgeons without spinal deformity training in fellowship.

---

63 *Le Huec JC, et al. Sagittal balance of the spine. European Spine Journal 28:1889-1905, 2019.*

Spinal Deformity - Cervical Scoliosis and Other Disorders of Spinal Malalignment

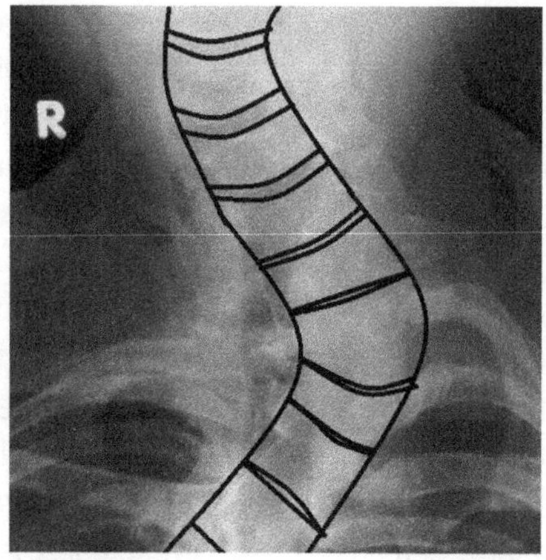

Figure 15-2. Cervical scoliosis, as seen in the above x-ray with the spine outlined. Most often, cervical scoliosis is very mild and is encountered during routine x-rays in older patients with neck pain. This scoliosis is typically a sign of neck compensation for a much larger thoracic or lumbar scoliosis, which is more frequently encountered. The body expends the least amount of energy when the center of gravity falls within the pelvis, and the head wants to be centered in the middle of the body. Fractures, scoliosis, and a number of other spinal conditions can cause a spinal deformity or scoliosis, leading to cervical compensation.

The Underlying Causes of Scoliosis Are Numerous And Impact Treatment Planning, Outcomes, and Complications

There are many causes of scoliosis. To treat it surgically, ie., decompress a nerve and fuse the spine, without understanding why the scoliosis occurred can have drastic consequences. Experience and practical knowledge in the treatment and management of scoliosis is just as important as a surgeon's training experience. Many conditions that cause painful spinal deformities do not always improve with surgery, or can continue to get worse, unless the underlying condition is not managed properly. Parkinson's disease, neuromuscular disorders, and even discrepancies in limb length (one leg longer than the other), can result in a failure to achieve satisfactory surgical goals for the patient.

While knowledge base does not translate into surgical skills, preoperative surgical planning and identification of the numerous causes of deformity are critical in successful outcomes. Surgical treatment are the most technically challenging in spinal surgery and the published technical complication rates are relatively greatest. Understanding the appropriate perioperative care for these patients can mean all the difference in achieving a positive outcome.

Overall, no major training differences exist between orthopedic and neurologic surgeons with regard to the most common causes of neck pain, which are cervical spinal degenerative conditions. In fact, a fairly recent query of the American College of Surgeon's National Surgical Quality Improvement Program Database found no difference between the two specialties in terms of 30-day readmission, surgical site infection, and mortality. Close to 10,000 patients were assessed in this study.[64] More specifically, the impact of training and clinical outcomes by neurosurgical or orthopedic-trained spine surgeons was evaluated, finding no significant differences between complications, readmissions, and revisions in spinal surgery.[65] The literature is fairly consistent on this in North America. If you have a degenerative spinal condition, you are in more than capable hands, irrespective of which office and specialty that you choose to go to.

---

64 *McCutcheon BA. Thirty-Day Perioperative Outcomes in Spinal Fusion by Specialty Within the NSQIP Database. Spine. 40(14):2015.*

65 *Mabud T et al. Complications, readmissions, and revisions for spine procedures performed by orthopedic surgeons versus neurosurgeons: A retrospective, longitudinal study. Clin Spine Surg. 30(10):E1376-E1381, 2017.*

16 What Are the Roles of the Spine Surgeon In Neck Pain Care?

With regards to degenerative conditions of the spine the traditional role of the spine surgeon has historically been to evaluate cadidates for spinal surgery after a trial of nonsurgical therapies and a basic diagnostic workup. Due to the rapidly growing complexity of the spinal care subfocus in tandem with tremendous population growth, many spinal surgeons have joined other spine specialists in the process of evaluating patients with acute pain, reviewing imaging and other diagnostic testing previously obtained, and helping patients develop a plan for care that is aligned with the patient's goals.

The majority of disc herniations, cervical muscle strain, and episodes of acute neck pain due to a degenerative spinal problem will spontaneously improve without intervention— again, this is assuming that there are no other variables that raise any flags, prompting a more urgent workup (see *red flags* chapter above).

Often, some spinal degenerative conditions may cause severe and disabling pain despite most nonsurgical therapies. For a number of other reasons, at the discretion of your primary care physician, a patient may be referred to a spinal surgeon for an evaluation in their clinic for surgery.[66] While this can be anxiety provoking, often patients are referred to spinal surgeons by their primary care physician because they are more comfortable with a spinal surgeon that they have developed a positive relationship with to facilitate the discussion around recently obtained imaging. In the event that it took some time to see this provider, a second referral can occur if the treatment required is not offered at the specialty spine clinic (such as an injection). This is very common since a referral to a surgeon in this instance may not always mean that surgery is needed.

66 For education related to acute pain, see the section, where can I go for immediate pain relief?

Abridged List of Common Services Offered by a Spinal Surgeon*

Urgent Evaluation (for diagnosis and treatment)
Surgical Treatment (eg. discectomy)
Referral for Physical Therapy
Minimally-invasive Surgical Options
Epidural Steroid Injections
Other Targeted Pain Injections
Spinal Cord Stimulation
Vertebroplasty
Referral to Another Specialist (other diagnotic testing): Neurologist, Orthopedic Surgeon, Diagnostic Injections, etc...

Always Confirm Services Prior to Scheduling An Appointment

Dramatic changes have occurred in the way that analgesic medications are prescribed, and therefore it is very important to diligently plan ahead. First, in many instances, patients are required (by insurance) to see their primary care physician/provider (PCP) first for acute pain, prior to obtaining a specialist.[67] When that

67 *That is, unless one is uninsured, or in the unlikely event that one decides to pay out of pocket, or has a form of insurance called a preferred provider organization, or PPO, where a primary care physician does not need to be selected and a referral is not needed in order to see other pro-*

healthcare provider believes that a spinal problem requires an MRI to be obtained, a referral to a spinal surgeon might quickly follow, as some providers find this to be more efficient, as often the management of some degenerative findings are less well defined. This initial visit will focus on an assessment and developing a care plan, which can often be referrals to other offices. This is a highly variable process, and often details like these can be obtained with a phone call. On the other hand, some physicians might not be limited by long wait times for patients and may have the resources to meet again to follow-up and discuss the results.

In other regions, some patients have to travel distances of greater than 60 miles to reach an appointment. When you are requesting to see a 'local' spine specialist that your primary care physician is unfamiliar with, it would be very important to determine from the destination office what is typically accomplished for new patients on the first visit.

Determining what to expect from the first visit and the list of services offered before making an appointment is very helpful; This is to prevent unnecessarily prolonging the time for a patient to obtain a diagnosis and/or relieve pain. If the initial appointment is mainly at the behest of the specialist who ordered the imaging, then that specialist should atleast be able to have the MRI in advance and provide an explanation of the findings and any further care plans. A spinal surgeon can review the imaging and discuss the nonsurgical treatment options, and in the case of some, the surgical options which are discussed in the final section of this book.

---

viders in the network, regardless of specialty. In the context of Medicare, the official Medicare site does explain the types of plans available, including the PPO. https://www.medicare.gov/sign-up-change-plans/types-of-medicare-health-plans/specialists-referrals-in-medicare-advantage-plans

Opiate Prescribing and Pain Management

The prescribing of pain medication varies from practice to practice. Overall, it is increasingly more difficult to get pain medication with the goal to prevent substance abuse and death. In 2018, there were over 67,000 deaths in a single year attributed to prescription opiate abuse. Typically, analgesics are prescribed for an agreed upon time period that would be deemed reasonable for the patient to transfer pain management and prescribing over to a new practice. The duration is dependent on clinic or healthcare guidelines, state guidelines, and other regional concerns.

Due to the opiate prescribing restrictions, many clinics may not or choose not to prescribe opiates for new patients or patients not requiring surgery. If it is determined that one meets the prescribing requirements at a practice, a pain management specialist referral could be given, and from that point, one might have to wait a long duration before obtaining a controlled pain medication. This can result in signifcant delay while one transitions between practices, which is a common problem as many pain management practices have closed in the past several years (see pain management,and opiate sections).

Pain management and social policy is a complex issue that is unable to be fully addressed in a handbook such as this. The environment is changing and it is confusing. Therefore, the biggest piece of advice the author can give is to call a facility prior to scheduling an appointment, determine the wait time, state one's needs/goals/expectations, and determine the clinics policies and expectations. This could save you months of wasted time. Specifically, determine the office's pain prescribing policy so as not to be left with any gaps in pain coverage.

Bring Your Records to every visit

Patients that take an active role in their healthcare are generally the most satisfied. It is important to note that being referred to see a physician does not automatically mean that the office that you were visiting has access to your entire healthcare history and all records that are associated with it, regardless if it is electronic or not. Sometimes, when you are referred to an office within the same healthcare system, the electronic medical record (EMR) software allows access to your physician for them to record and view these records. Also, they can add to your records and imformation from outside the network can be download (eg. an MRI), and paperwork be scanned (eg. a printed record from an outpatient lab). The end result is to help limit unnecessarily repeating studies and to help improve your quality of care.

But not all offices will be able to access that information. Some EMR systems have software, training, and maintenance costs (databases and expanded personell requirements) that are only affordable by large healthcare systems, and not with s mall private practices. Regardless of the size, without a signed consent from the practice one has an appointment with (unless you consented for all providers in a healthcare system) they will not be able to request any records. The bottom line is, the more complete the healthcare record that you bring with you, the better the care can be for you.

One misconception is that referring practices will automatically send all medical records. This is not always the case and it can be very tedious to confirm on the phone that all nececssary records were sent. First, the process to obtain records begins with your active participation where written consent is provided by you (usually a practice has a form for you to complete) to initiate the release of your medical records to specific parties. At the present time, the most efficient process is to make copies of all of your medical records and to make them available to each new practice. This is mainly to help You avoid the need to reschedule an appointment, or to have another duplicate test obtained as studies can are often become lost when practices close, patients move, or there records become increasingly more complex over a span of years.

SECTION III

SPINE IMAGING EXPLAINED

17 What's the Best Imaging For The Neck (X-ray, CT, or MRI)?

Spinal imaging has grown to become an essential component of modern neck pain management. In the following sections, the most common imaging studies will be discussed, and how they differ from each other, and why more than one type might be necessary. Spinal imaging is a catch-all term referring to any test that provides information about a patient's normal and abnormal anatomy. As healthcare becomes more specialized, independent pathways of care and recommendations for imaging studies are being implemented for various causes of neck pain. For example, episodes of acute neck pain in association with a sport's related injury, or a trauma, or prior spine surgery, will undergo a different imaging workup. These causes of neck pain will certainly undergo a different institutional pathway for workup and a patient who got out of bed with the feeling of sharp neck pain, without any other worrisome features. Most people with neck pain with less than a three month history of neck pain and no significant past medical history (see red flags) should attempt, if at all possible, to avoid non-invasive and advanced diagnostic measures for neck pain, as the majority of patients with neck pain have spontaneous relief.[68]

The reason cited is usually that an MRI under the standard protocols does not identify muscle strain, the most common cause of neck pain. Moreover, the cervical MRI does little more than shift the clinical focus of the patient and staff towards unfounded and needless treatments for degenerative spinal disease — spondylosis, disc herniations, and disc degeneration— These pathologies may have been present long before the onset of pain. This possibility is underscored by studies finding a high incidence of degenerative conditions of the spine in volunteers without a history of neck pain or injury. Again, this ultimately raises the complexity and cost, and also the risks that come with more frequently performed invasive non-surgical treatments. Most often muscle strain will evantually recover, just as any pulled muscle does. On the otherhand, if the pain is so severe that it is not possible to concentrate, not relieved by over the counter analgesics, and even potentially unsafe to go to work, these of course represent a subset of patients where further workup would be prudent.

---

68 *Patients with neurologic deficits such as weakness, numbness, extremity pain, and other red flag symptoms should obtain an urgent evaluation. This will most likely include an MRI if the examiner feels that these symptoms are related. See the section on red flag symptoms with any additional questions.*

The Basic Spinal Imaging Tests are the X-ray, CT, and MRI

In the following chapters of this imaging section, Important imaging regarding the X-ray, CT, and MRI will be discussed regarding the strengths and weakness of each spinal imaging test. Overall, the MRI is the most sensitive for identifying causes of cervical degenerative disease as it is the only test that can clearly show soft tissues such as the nerves and disc. MRI is in fact so much more helpful for detecting nerve compression and evaluating disc disease/spondylosis, that several issues arise.

Magnetic Resonance Imaging and False Positives

The most detailed imaging studies, the MRI, provides unparalleled detail of the soft tissues in the body. Several challenges to diagnosis arise from higher resolution. The first problem is that false positive and negative findings do still occur. A false positive test is one that erroneously gives a positive result in patients that do not have the disease in question, while a false negative erroneously does not show the disease being evaluated for.[69] The next challenge will be the interpretation of the MRI, where variability does exist from one observer to the next as to how an MRI is interpreted. The last challenge is the identification of incidental spinal

---

69 *A false positive test is classically used for a test that only has positive or negative finding, and not for a test that requires interpretation. However, when the test is ordered to find the underlying cause of the specific painful symptoms, the MRI test can be summarized as having a yes/no answer. A false positive result in this instance means that the MRI found an underlying cause, when in fact, no underlying cause of pain was identified. Essentially, this is the incidental finding.*

pathology not causing the pain, as mentioned above, which complicates the picture.

The majority of patients that undergo an MRI of the spine for acute neck pain will be over 30 years old, and therefore, inter alia will have some kind of natural process of spondylosis, ie. degenerative disc disease (Fig 17-1). Patients are oftened surprised to learn that the initial finding of a disc herniation may include disc bulges, extrusions, protrusions, sequestrations, annular fissures, spurs, spondylosis, spondylolisthesis, and facet cysts are not substantial enough in most cases to link to low back pain without further workup. Additionally, these are findings that can change very little over time, or rapidly arise, and therefore cannot be reliably linked to any specific event.[70]

---

70 *see incidental findings, at the end of the imaging section.*

* *Numerous reports study various aspects of the incidence of common cervical MRI findings, and are included in the bibliography at the end. It is important to know that every choice made by the researchers as to how to conduct the study influences the results.*

Frequency of Cervical MRI Findings in Volunteer Patients with and without Neck Pain

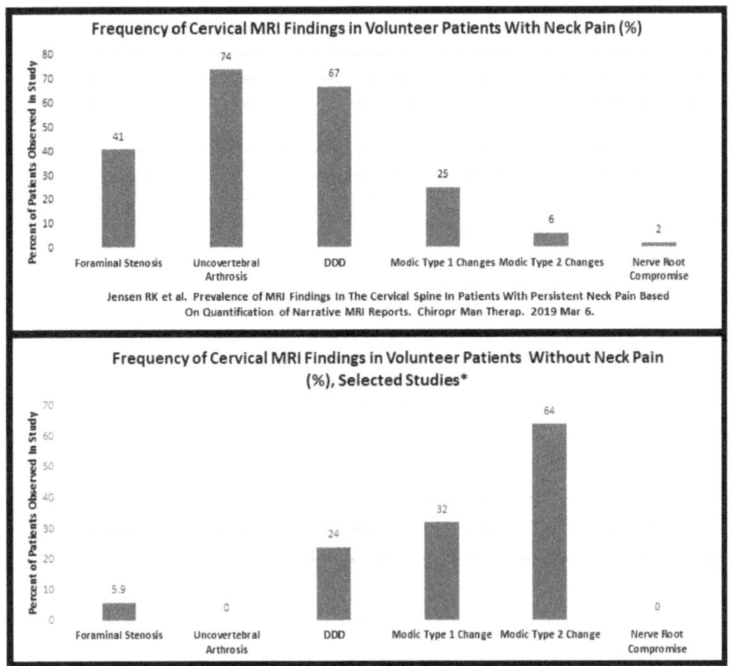

Figure 17-1. Common cervical MRI findings as reported in one study (top graph) are compared with findings in studies consisting of patients without neck pain (bottom graph). With the comparison limited to these two studies, the conclusions are limited. However, degenerative disc disease and the associated modic changes are still frequent findings in both groups of patients. Patients with foraminal stenosis and arthritic changes (listed as uncovertebral arthrosis above) in the facet joint were more likely to have neck pain. Note how 75% of patients with neck pain had uncovertebral arthrosis, a finding not found in patients without neck pain. Keep in mind that these studies merely show an association and do not definitively prove that certain features found on MRI cause neck pain.

Imaging and Red Flags

As mentioned previously 'Red flag Symptoms' are less defined for neck pain as compared with low back pain. However, if the same set of red flags are present in the context of neck pain, the same concerns exist and the clinical recommendations are in effect the same. **Imaging may be necessary in the event of weakness, difficulty walking, abnormal bowel or bladder function, trauma, osteoporosis, a history of cancer, LBP or neck pain that is worse at night, fever, and ongoing treatment for an active infection or a history of recreational drug abuse.** The most appropriate imaging study varies. The MRI is the most sensitive of the diagnostic tests, and often results in the greatest degree of findings, but this may not be what is required for each situation. Any decision making to obtain imaging requires an order by a healthcare provider, this also can include a chiropractor in most states.[71] MRIs are essential for diagnosing nerve compression.

If at all possible, and you have not met any 'red flag conditions' it is important to avoid obtaining an MRI in the first several months of neck pain due to the excellent chance of spontaneous improvement. MRI imaging usually will find something, which can then become a point of unnecessary focus. Many clinicians are going to

---

71 *For a review of the chiropractic scope of practice by state see: Chang M. The chiropractic scope of practice in the United States: A Cross-sectional survey. 37(6):363-376, 2014.*

find it hard to ignore the results of an MRI in the absence of another concrete diagnosis. Muscle strain and even spinal causes of pain, such as discogenic pain do not have a reliable method of diagnosis. Even if the clinician is convinced that these findings are not the cause of the pain, it is still difficult in many cases to have a high degree of certainty one way or the other and therefore many patients will have a hard time convincing themselves. Again, just because there is a "finding" on an MRI, doesn't mean it is causing pain!

Recall that research studies have identified a very high frequency of spinal degenerative conditions diagnosed by MRI in volunteers without any history of neck or back problems. This finding has been repeated again and again. Correlation does note equal causation.

18 When Should I Get X-Rays?

When X-rays are generated, they are focused through a tube, and a relative picture is created on the basis that radiation travels through varrying density tissues in the body and that creates a gradient, or a picture, which is then captured on a plate.[72] This was originally captured on film in order to create the imaging study. This was later placed with a mechanism to digitally capture the image, without film. Decades of study pertaining to the appearance of spinal anatomy on plain films (an x-ray) and the characterization of normal anatomy and spinal diseases makes x-ray studies clinically useful for specific indications, even after the widespread adoption

72 *For a more detailed explanation of x-rays, and their generation, this website contains in-depth descriptions with illustration: "https://www.radiologymasterclass.co.uk/tutorials/physics/x-ray_physics_production" Accessed May 20, 2020.*

of the CT and MRI. Always, the quality of the information obtained by the imaging is dependent on the provider and what reason the test was ordered, as well as other factors such as the technician obtaining the study and the skilled interpreter who 'reads' the imaging and creates a report, the radiologist.

Most degenerative conditions of the spine that produces painful neck and extremity symptoms are doing so via compression of a nerve root. Nerve roots are not shown on x-rays, because they are not dense enough. Foraminal stenosis, or the narrowing of the channels where nerve roots exit the spine, may be caused by growth of the facet joints (which also causes neck pain). Other structures that appear on x-ray due to their bony composition include osteophytes (spurs) but the significance of these structures cannot be assessed without demonstrating that compression of nerve tissue is occuring on an MRI. Even if an x-ray gave the patient the impression that there was isolated one-level cervical disc disease and spondylosis with some foraminal stenosis, which implicates that there is nerve compression, an MRI is still used in most cases to confirm that there is in fact compression, and that there isn't compression at adjacent levels, as well as assess a number of other clinical factors. Surgical planning very commonly includes an MRI, as it will show indirectly in three-dimensional space where the point of compression is located and complicating factors such as the extent of foraminal stenosis and the type of disc herniations, the presence of spinal cord compression, etc...

X-rays Provide a Limited Assessment of Soft Tissues

Disc herniations are usually soft, and x-rays are of little benefit to evaluate soft tissue. They also do not assess the contents of the disc space. The degree of disc degeneration would only be implied by the loss of disc height and the presence of bone changes and osteophytes. Regarding bone, MRI and X-ray are also less sensitive than CT in evaluation of bone, including fractures,[73] and even more so with patients with lower bone density (osteoporotic) which makes interpretation of small, linear, non-displaced fractures relatively more challenging with plain films. Since an x-ray only provides a 2-dimensional picture on a flat x-ray film, at least two x-ray studies with perpendicular trajectories through the same the same three dimensional space are required to extrapolate the three-dimensional nature of the spine. Even with two x-rays, there is no comparison to the degree of detail generated from a CT. Nonetheless, there are many important uses for radiographs (x-ray studies/ plain films/radiographs all mean the same thing to a layman).

While x-rays still have their place in spinal care— as an intial test, they have incredible limitations for acute neck pain. Recall again that with uncomplicated acute neck pain, it is recommended that imaging studies not be obtained to begin with. They are still very useful as a screening tool to evaluate a patient's spinal alignment, evaluate spinal surgical instrumentation, and a general evaluation tool for trauma, infection, limb pain, atypical pain, osteoporosis, and degenerative conditions, to a name a few. Additionally, they are inexpensive and easy enough to be obtained periodically through time to evaluate for any chronic changes that may be occurring.

---

73 *Antevil JL et al. Spiral computed tomography for the initial evaluation of spine trauma: A new standard of care? J Trauma. 61(2)382-7:2006.*

Selected Indications For Plain Cervical Spine Radiographs[74]

- Evaluate for fracture
- Assess regional alignment
- Assess and measure cervical deformity and scoliosis
- Evaluate spinal surgery instrumentation
- Assessment of degenerative changes
- Evaluate for bony destruction by tumors and infection

Of the studies, they are the least expensive to obtain and frequently do not require prior approval to obtain and are found in imaging centers in many practices. However, while cervical radiographs are still an important tool, they are have a relatively lower diagnostic value compared to an MRI or CT.

---

74 *For a review of imaging indications, discussion of cases and example imaging, specialized types x-ray studies, radiopaedia.org is an excellent online educational resource: https://radiopaedia.org/articles/cervical-spine-series?lang=us*

What is Bone Density Scanning and Bone Densitometry?

Bone density scanning/densitometry[75] takes advantage of the concept that as bone becomes more dense (increases in mineral density), less x-rays penetrate through the spine (Figure 18-1). The amount of x-rays that make it through the spine can be measured and compared to the average. This measurement provides an indirect estimate of bone density.

The World Health Organization defined osteoporosis as a T Score of more than 2.5 standard deviations below the mean bone density for young adults. This cutoff should be looked at as a gradient where the lower the T score, the greater the lifetime risk of additional fractures.[76]

Dual energy absorptiometry, or, a DEXA scan, uses data obtained from x-ray beams with relatively high and low energy to provide accurate information and is needed to diagnose osteoporosis.[77] Women in the US are at an elevated risk for osteoporosis and osteopenia. As a point of preventative care, this is one of the most overlooked aspects of health care and untreated osteoporosis is a serious fracture risk in the elderly.

---

75 *This is also simplified. For more detail: https://www.aapm.org/meetings/03AM/pdf/9873-13152.pdf*
Another excellent explanation is on one cleveland clinic medical education website:
https://www.clevelandclinicmeded.com/medicalpubs/ccjm/Jan06/watts.htm#:~:text=The%20WHO%20working%20group%20selected,of%20fracture%20at%20these%20sites.

76 *Marshall D, Johnell O, Wedel H. Meta-analysis of how well measures of bone mineral density predict occurrence of osteoporotic fractures. BMJ 1996; 312:1254–1259.*

77 *See related info for other less common radiologic tests of bone absorptiometry: https://www.aapm.org/meetings/03AM/pdf/9873-13152.pdf*

The Bone Densitometry Machine Uses X-rays To Approximate Mineralization Of The Bone And Help Identify Patients At Risk From Spine, Hip, and Other Long Bone Fractures

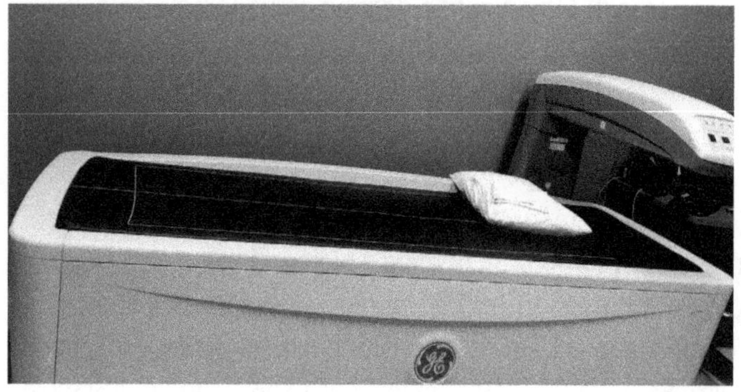

Figure 18-1. Bone Densitometry Machine (Seen in photo: Scanner manufactured by General Electric Company, Norwalk, CT).

19 **When Should I Get a CT ?**

It is amazing that the CT scan (computed tomography) is rapidly approaching it's fifty-year anniversary of valuable clinical service. The CT is very valuable, in that it provides tremendous information in three dimensions, whereas an x-ray of the spine provides some information in 2-dimensions. The costs of this technology is an increase in radiation exposure. For neck pain, as well will show below, that this is generally a poor study, and exposes very sensitive structures such as the brain and thyroid to needless radiation, when an MRI is a superior study to asssess for most causes of acute radicular (or even axial) neck pain.

Imagine using information obtained from 360 degrees, where multiple scans are obtained while an xray machine is spun in a tube in a concentric circle around the patient, scanning periodically. Using this information and innovative calculations,[78] a map of three

78 *Called the Fourier Transform, the mathematical technique has many applications both medican and nonmedical. For those that are inter-*

dimensional space can be made from this. CT scans rely on radiation and can be used to obtain three-dimensional imaging, whereas x-rays produce a two-dimensional image. Technically, all imaging is produced on a flat surface, and therefore it is a two dimensional image, but more three dimensional representations (cross-sections) are directly provided. Spinal surgeons, the CT scan is excellent for evaluating trauma patients and as an occasional guide for surgical decisionmaking which is beyond the scope of this book.

A CT scan is a similar appearing machine to an MRI, except a much easier process to tolerate, as it is much quicker, quieter, and less confined and the scanner is less confining of a space, relative to MRI (Fig. 19-1). You lay on a mobile bed, that will move you briefly through a hollow tube, in which the x-ray emitter and detectors rotate through to send and measure the x-rays, respectively. Unfortunately, as an assessment tool for most degenerative disc pathology and degenerative conditions of the spine, the CT scan is not ideal to detect soft tissue problems. Another drawback from using these studies for the attempt to provide a surrogate assessment, is the exposure of radiation to the patient, and risk of cancer (Fig. 19-2). An MRI is the preferred imaging study for the evaluation of these conditions. Once again, CT scans of the spine excel at evaluating fractures, calcified disc herniations, and other conditions that involve changes to, or involving tissues of high density, namely bone.

---

ested, it is described in the aptly titled book, The Fourier Transform and It's Applications, by Ronald N. Bracewell.

Computed Tomography (CT)

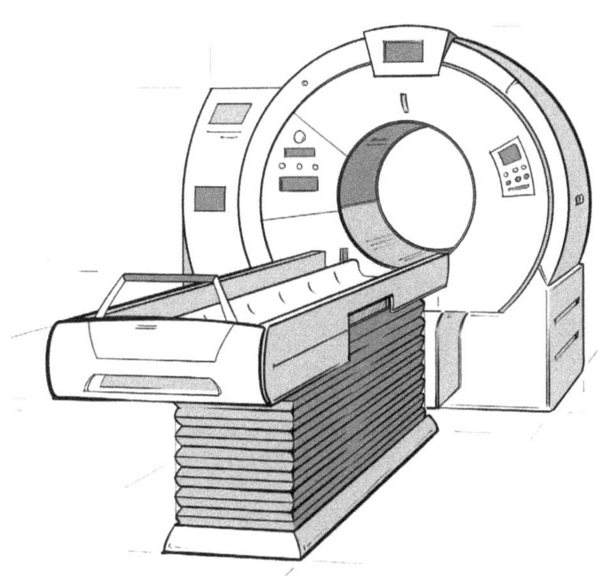

Figure 19-1. Computed Tomography ('CT Scan') For most spine imaging studies, the process of the table passing briefly passing through the center results in high quality imaging in minutes or less. (Artist Illustration, From 'The Low Back Pain Book')

How Much Radiation Am I Exposed To From A CT Scans Compared To A Chest X-ray?

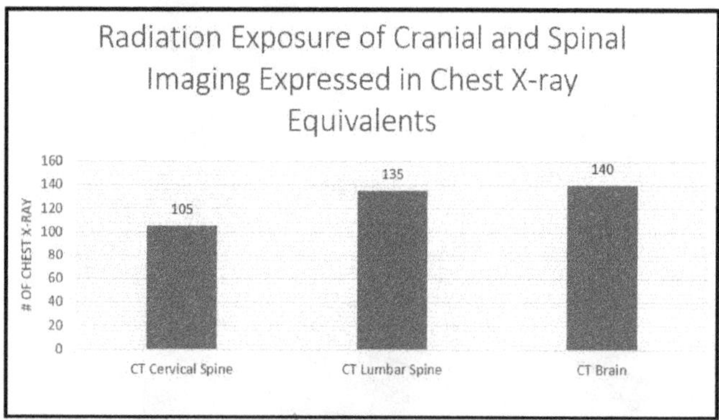

Figure 19-2. Number of X-rays, where dose = 0.02 mSv/ average chest x-ray.[79] Keep in mind that these numbers vary across studies and protocols. But the general message is, CT scans produce three-dimensional imaging using information obtained from many simppler two-dimensional images.

---

79 *Brix et al. Eur Radiol 2003;13:1979.*

20 **What Is An MRI (Magnetic Resonance Imaging)?**

MRI (Magnetic resonance imaging) is an imaging technique that provides detailed images of a patient's anatomy. The essential components include a large electromagnet generating a magnetic field— strong enough to influence the orientation of the magnetic fields of the small hydrogen atoms in our body, while laying in the scanner (Fig 20-1). The second and essential part of the test involves radio waves being transmitted and received across the patient. These signals are what is used to make the images. This process has been refined over the years to improve the diagnostic value of the studies by increasing resolution, and decreasing the time that a patient spends in the scanner. MRIs do not rely on ionizing radiation and do not use X-rays.

MRI Utilizes Hydrogen In Our Body

As we mentioned, an MRI can temporarily align positive charges (protons) in the body. Since water concentrations vary throughout the body, when the MRI aligns the charges, radio waves are pulsed through the body to put the protons out of alignment. The time for the protons to realign with the magnetic field and any energy released varies by the tissue type. Refinements to the technique over time have allowed for very detailed anatomical pictures of the spine to be obtained.[80]

An MRI provides excellent imaging of the condition of the intervertebral disc as disc degeneration is a process of water loss from the disc space. Recall that the disc contains proteoglycans that hold several times its volume in water molecules, which contain two hydrogen atoms. Now, the lack of water content is one common feature that explains why they are poorly visualized on MRI. Bone, or more accurately, the denser cortical bone on the surface of bone, dense arthritic surfaces, have a relatively poor blood supply, or none altogether, and therefore contain very little water, which in turn does not show up well on MRI. The cancellous bone, which is deep to the cortical bone, contains blood vessels and marrow, and is easier to visualize on MRI due to the blood supply. One reason for this is that blood is 92% water, another factor that influences the appearance of a substance like blood on MRI is the

---

80 *Interestingly, while the MRI scanner relies on proton (1H), in research, hydrogen is not the only element that can be evaluated. However, it makes the most sense since water is about 2/3 of our mass. An odd atomic number or odd number of neutrons have a nuclear magnetic moment (which is the strength and orientation of the magnetic field). For a more complete description of how the MRI machine works, see MRI physics, by Andrew Murphy and Ray Ballinger in https://radiopaedia.org/articles/mri-physics?lang=us.*

type of sequence, which is generally the manner and frequency in which the radio waves are pulsed, producing unique measurements that allow for an MRI study that has a greater diagnostic value.[81] Blood is an interesting substance with a variable appearance on MRI, largely due to the iron-containing moleculre hemoglobin, which, as an oxygen carrier, changes the magentic field properties with the presence or absence of oxygen. Another factor that influences MRI appearance is the presence of blood outside of the blood vessel, which can occur with a bruise or blood clot. In a blood clot, the concentration and ratios of different types of hemoglobin molecules impact the magnetic field of hemoglobin and the presence of oxygen bound to hemoglobin (affects the magnetic properties of the iron in hemoglobin).

Disc Degeneration

The process of disc degeneration results in a gradual loss of water, making it ideal to be evaluated by an MRI study. During adolescence, the disc is water rich, containing a unique signal. With degeneration, this signal is gradually changing.[82] While a CT scan cannot reliably and clearly show the boundaries of a nerve root, spinal cord, or disc herniation, the MRI is able to show all of these things as well as inflammation and swelling in a nerve or the spinal cord. One of the hallmarks of inflammation is the process of abnormal blood vessel permeability[83] and new blood vessel formation,

---

81 *Murphy A and Gaillard F. MRI sequences (overview) in https://radiopaedia.org/articles/mri-sequences-overview?lang=us*

82 *A full characterization of the changes on a biologic level is summarized in the preceding disc degeneration chapter, and in the following chapter on MRI grading of disc degeneration.*

83 *Askenase MH. Stages of the inflammatory response in pathology and tissue repair after intracerebral hemorrhage. Semin Neurol. 36(3):288-297, 2016.*

which leads to increases in water concentration in the tissues. Water is increased in the region of inflammation, which explains why a bruised tissue becomes enlarged after an injury. MRI is particularly sensative to inflammation.

Magnetic Resonance Imaging

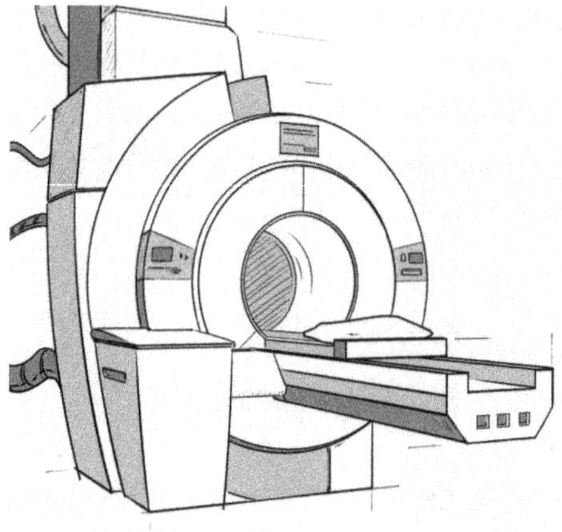

Figure 20-1. The MRI Scanner (From The Low Back Pain Guide, 2019). The MRI scanning bed retracts into a more confined space for a period of minutes to hours. The MRI scanner is loud, and patients typically wear ear protection. For patients with difficulty in confined spaces (claustrophobia, anxiety, severe pain while laying flat, etc...), this may often require some type of mild sedation.

21 How Can I Better Understand My MRI Report?

The spinal MRI report is almost always concerning for patients, because it is uncommon for an adult to see a report that says 'normal'. Before describing aspects of the MRI report, some background information is needed regarding the physician who specializes in writing this report. A diagnostic neuroradiologist specializes in medical imaging of the nervous system. This is a subspeciality within radiology. A neuroradiology fellowship requires two years of additional training, which is after the 4 year diagnostic radiology residency, which is also after a 1 year internship in medicine, which is still part of residency. Let's not also forget the additional 4 years of undergraduate college in any subject and 4 years of medical school. On average, that is 15 years of school, unless one encounters one of many physicians with additional degrees, such as those with masters degrees and doctorates. A 'PhD, MD', the 'physician-scientist', and is a truly dedicated individual. This is someone who after all of this time, to become a physician, decides to take an additional 3-4 years of time to master an area of laboratory research, obtain a doctorate to dedicate themselves to advancing medical knowledge (eg. in biology, biochemistry, or really in any number of fields). Those that do this mainly have the desire to improve the quality of medicine through clinical research, more than for any other reason. That's close to 20 years of education after high school. This extensive training requirement should illustrate that interpreting imaging appropriately cannot be done by any individual with a book or textbook bought online, and definitely not in these general lessons.

Certainly, even if one fooled themselves into thinking they could read their own MRI, it cannot be appreciated and understood at the same critical level that these gifted individuals spent so many years getting certified for, and then gathering experience in clinical practice. This would be like the author writing editorials on modern art.- If the reader has had the fortune to go to the Museum of Modern Art in New York, he or she will vividly grasp that without an art background, much of modern art is hard to understand. Modern art may possibly be easier to understand than an MRI without a background in spinal imaging. That approximates the scale of attempting to briefly interpret an MRI. However, anatomy and MRI atlases of the spine are available if you are eager to learn. As one will find out, a small amount of background reading in medicine can go a long way to alleviate anxiety by gaining a slightly better understanding of the medical processes. And even still, without expert guidance and a residency training, learning to interpret radiology, especially in a short time for the practical purpose of understanding and self-diagnosis is very unrealistic.

MRI Report: A More Reasonable Goal Than MRI Interpretation

Fortunately, the task of improving one's understanding of the cervical MRI report is possible, especially since the majority of the findings are related to spinal degenerative conditions. One has to keep in mind that again, there is a limitation when attempting to independently determine the clinical signifance of the finding. For example, a neuroradiologist states in a hypothetical MRI report that, "at the level of C7-C8, there is a left-sided disc-osteophyte complex causing left neuroforaminal stenosis." The significance of this finding with a patient with opposite-sided right hand pain, or pain radiating into the left shoulder is not known. Ultimately, the easiest way to find out the significance (or lack thereof) of the report findings is to ask your physician. Otherwise, keep reading. There are a few general considerations. The first consideration is that most degenerative findings can be present in an MRI of patients without symptoms. The second is that neck pain can just as easily occur from any level of the spine, from muscle strain, or a number of other reasons, and without other information, an MRI isn't going to diagnose neck pain. The next consideration is that the side and level of the nerve compression must match the symptoms. Compression of the C8 nerve does not cause shoulder symptoms, but compression of the C5 nerve can (in most people). Also, many underlying orthopedic problems can cause hand or shoulder symptoms. So, it is important to keep in mind that an MRI is just imaging of the spine, and isn't going to tell one explicitly what the underlying process that is occurring, and it is important to avoid that mindset.

The MRI report is broken into several sections which are the same on every report, so understanding each section is helpful. The next undertaking is to undertand the terminology used in each section (eg. spondylosis, degenerative disc disease, etc.).[84]

Components Of The Radiology Report

- *Report header:* The report header is found at the top of the report and contains the name of the facility and address of where the study was performed. It usually contains a contact phone number as well.

- *Patient Identification Information:* Fairly self-explanatory but for the sake of completeness this section includes at least your name, date of birth, age, and usually a medical record number that is used by the facility storing your records which is often unique in the case of a private imaging facility.

- *Type Of Examination:* This is a brief title of the study being performed (e.g., 'CT lumbar spine, without contrast).

- *Clinical history:* The clinical history is usually kept to a minimum by software design and is not uncommon to see a two to three word-long description. For example, "back and leg pain, 3 months."

---

84 *It is important to realize that most people will not be able to understand or interpret their MRI report and should seek advice from a spinal healthcare expert. As previously mentioned, the biggest limiting factor is the incredible amount of time needed to be a radiologist.*

- *Comparisons:* Occasionally, when a complex study is repeated at the same facility, comparisons are made to ask ourselves, "Is there anything that has changed?" This is valuable for spinal problems as when symptoms change, it is important to ask if the spine has changed as well. This is especially helpful when comparing imaging with known issues and prior operationg. The reading radiologist will typically comment on the prior study, including the date from which the prior report was performed. Usually, the actual description of the comparison is reported at the end of the findings.

- *Technique*: Further description on how the exam was done is found in this section. If contrast was administered, that is also included here. Details included are the thickness of each image slice (distance between each image), and reformatted images that were included for analysis (eg. coronal and sagittal images).

- *Findings:* This is the main section of the report and details what the radiologist 'found'.

- *Impression:* This is a summary of the findings. The findings section will be quite lengthy and in this section the radiologist will provide a conclusion, often a diagnosis, and occasionally a differential diagnosis when the findings are not conclusive. Occasionally, recommendations of other helpful studies may be included.

- *Signature:* Containing the name of the radiologist who provided the report, with the date and time. This is often a digital signature.

- *Addendums:* Occasionally further information may be identified and added to a finalized and signed study- this will be included in the addendum.

- *Additional Attachments:* Additional attachments are often found at the end, and can include summaries of radiation exposure to the patient in the case of radiographs and other relevent studies, or other typical intake forms such as screening for relevent medical problems that may are a matter of patient safety during the study. Eg. Metallic implants prior to an MRI study, or intravenous contrast allergy. A review of systems by the technologist is study and facility specific. Other documents found include billing forms and a physician order for the imaging study.

22 **How Soon Do I Need An MRI?**

To date, for sudden-onset (acute) neck pain, without any other symptoms, an MRI is not usually required. Neither is a CT or X-ray, for that matter, except in certain circumstances which is usually at the discretion of your physician after a review of the complete clinical picture (eg. neck pain after a motor vehicle collision, raises the likelihood of major injury, as opposed to awaking up with neck pain and no other associated symptoms or relevant history).[85] Since most neck pain is due to paraspinal muscle strain and degenerative cervical spine conditions such as a soft disc herniation, this will not be seen adequately on a CT or an X-ray. On a cervical CT study, general comments are often made about the appearance of the disc in the cervical spine but the significance of the disc herniation, whether it be compressive, or causing significant stenosis

85 *There are some specific circumstances where management can change. Please see chapter 8, cervical red flag symptoms, for additional questions.*

cannot be made without an MRI. They most certainly will not be able to determine if nerve root or spinal cord compression is occurring for most disc herniations. CT studies are not a substitute for an MRI, but in practice, this is common. Recall that most neck pain spontaneously improves— To allow for that improvement to happen before too many tests and treatments can be ordered through the insurance carrier, companies require additional treatments to be attempted prior to obtaining an MRI. Most often, a primary care provider will evaluate the patient first, in order to evaluate for concerning conditions that warrant an early MRI.

MRI Reports and Disc Bulges

When neck pain correlates with additional symptoms, such as pain radiating down the arm, this can be very helpful in identifying the cervical level where the symptoms arise. This depends on where the disc herniation is located and where your pain is located (Fig. 22-1). Just remember, there are no absolutes! There are variations in patient dermatome locations, which are the regions of the skin that correlate to specific nerve roots. There are numerous examples in atlases and found online where variations in dermatome maps are encountered. Not all patients are wired the same way— This is just another of the many challenges with correlating nerve compression and painful symptoms (Fig. 22-2).[86]

86 *McAnany SJ et al, Oberserved Patterns of Cervical Radiculopathy: How Often Do They Differ From a Standard, "Netter Diagram" Distribution? Spine J. 2019 19(7):1137-1142.*

Cervical Nerve Root Compression/Radiculopathy: Frequent Sensory and Pain Complaints

Disc Herniation Level (nerve root compressed)	Complaints attributed to nerve compression
C4-C5 (C5)	Pain and sensory changes in the (lateral) upper arm and shoulder/ deltoid and bicep weakness.
C5-C6 (C6)	Pain and sensory changes in the outer forearm and thumb/ weakness flexing the elbow and pronating the forearm.
C6-C7 (C7)	Pain and sensory changes in the forearm and middle finger, often partial index and ring finger involvement/ extension of elbow and wrist.
C7-T1 (C8)	Pain and sensory changes in the (medial) ulnar forearm, little finger, and adjacent half of ring finger / grip strength weakness.
C7-T1 (T1)	Pain and sensory changes in the inner-aspect of the upper arm / hand intrinsic muscle strength.

Figure 22-1. Cervical radiculopathy and nerve root compression syndromes vary considerably. Often, patients may experience only some of the typical symptoms, or a pain pattern correlating to a different dermatome altogether. For example, C6 nerve compression with symptoms in the hand only (ie. thumb), or symptoms in the upper arm only, and some patients experience a pain that involves the upper chest (pectoralis muscle). Patients with cervical radiculopathy should consult their physician and discuss their symptoms, especially with the presence of weakness. One final consideration for seeing a physician promptly upon the onset of left arm and chest pain is the overlap with symptoms of a life threatening cardiac disease (see Chapter 8 for red flag symptoms section).

The Cervical Dermatome Map - One Variant

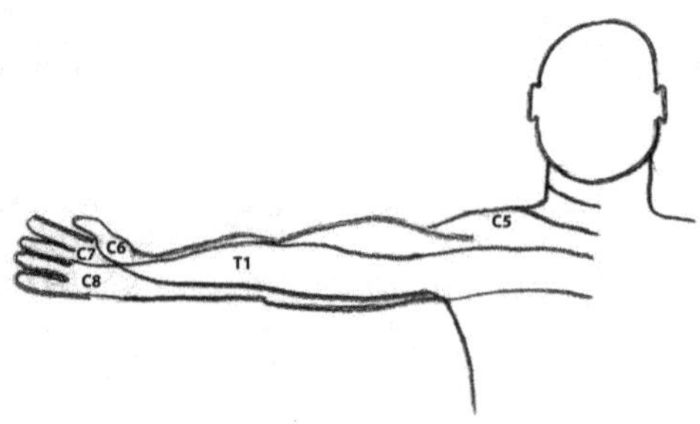

Figure 22-2. The cervical dermatome map corresponding to the above table. Note that this is just one of a few examples in circulation. The numbered nerve roots above correspond to one frequently report dermatome map. The differences between dermatome maps are most striking when the fingers are compared from one dermatome map to the next. This is due to individual variations in human anatomy from one person to the next, or due to inflammation of nearby nerve roots in close proximity to a disc. For example, a C5-6 disc herniation may compress the exiting C6 nerve, or in close proximity the (also called, traversing nerve root) C7 nerve root, passing nearby to exit at the C6-7 neural foramen.

What Are The Strengths of an MRI?

This is what you obtain when you are looking for the majority of problems in the spine. MRIs are helpful for disc disease and are the single most important study for the diagnosis and evaluation of a herniated disc.

What if an MRI Can Not Be Safely Obtained?

An MRI cannot always be obtained safely. Some patients have metallic foreign bodies, incompatible surgical implants, and other medical reasons preventing someone from laying flat and motionless for the duration of the lengthy test, which includes severe back pain, claustrophobia, to name a few. One very common contraindication to an MRI is with an incompatible pacemaker. All efforts should be made to confirm with a radiologist that an MRI is not possible. It is surprising that certain centers vary in terms of MRI compatibility, but they do.

The CT Myelogram

The alternative study to the MRI that can be obtained is the **CT myelogram.** A CT myelogram provides evidence of spinal cord compression in an indirect manner, which is less valuable than an MRI, but in some instances it is the only acceptable option. A CT myelogram still relies on a CT scan, and therefore exposure to radiation. The concept of a CT is that it is a test that indirectly shows compression of the nerves or spinal cord. The first step is a lumbar puncture (Fig. 22-3) where contrast is injected into the lumbar spine, and mixed with spinal fluid. This makes spinal fluid appear brighter on a CT scan. In absence of compression of the nerves or spinal cord (eg. by a disc herniation), this bright CSF is easily seen to flow around the cord, and part of the nerve roots, which appear darker than the fluid.

Disc herniations indent the covering of the nerves and the spinal cord, and can be seen indirectly, by the impression made (Fig 21-3, letter A). This fluid is made in the brain and continuous from the brain to the lumbar spine.

The (CT) Myelogram Principle

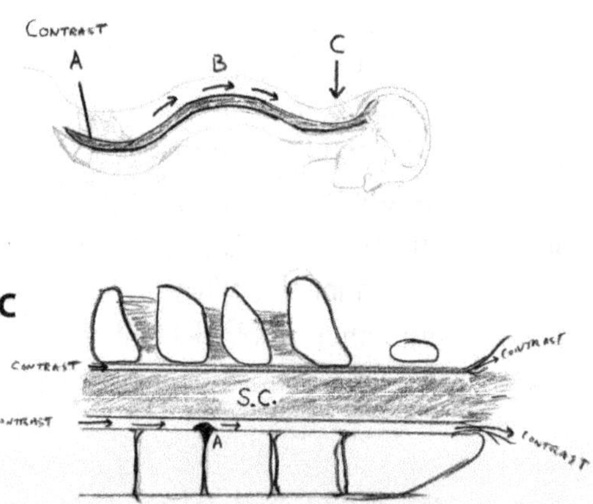

Figure 22-3. CT Myelogram. Contrast is injected into the spinal canal (emphasized in top figure) in a sterile lumbar puncture (A). The fluid flows in the direction of the head, which is facilitated by tilting the procedure table. The patient then undergoes a CT scan a few minutes later after the injection. The resulting imaging of the cervical spine, for example, shows a bright space (arrows in image 'C') around the spinal cord (S.C.). Disc herniations are visible in regions with a discontinuity in the smooth bright contours where contrast wound normally be found-ie over the disc space (A). This is a form of indirect visualization of stenosis (the 'negative').

The technique of a CT myelogram is performed by an experienced physician or a technician under supervision, usually a neuroradiologist, or interventional radiologist. A needle is placed into the lumbar spinal canal, entering the dura and end up in the resevoir where the CSF is located. Since iodinated contrast dye is injected during a lumbar spinal puncture, allergies to iodine can make this a very troublesome procedure, and can even preclude someone from having this test. Having severe lumbar spinal stenosis, prior lumbar spinal surgery, and other conditions can prevent the successful visualization of the cervical spine with adequate contrast. The capabilities and ability vary from institution to institution in terms of a facility's ability to accomodate a patient's unique medical and surgical issues. A lumbar puncture carries the risk of a spinal headache, which is caused by drainage of spinal fluid out of the needle puncture site over the spinal canal. To limit this risk, patients are kept flat for a few hours to limit the pressure gradient across this puncture site and allow it to close appropriately. Spinal headaches are very painful and fortunately relatively uncommon.

This study is the same, regardless of the location of interest, lumbar myelogram, thoracic myelogram, or cervical myelogram, the injection is usually lumbar and the CT is performed over the region of interest. This study may be superior to an MRI in patients that have had extensive prior spinal surgery— Very often, the metallic implants distort the signal from the magnetic field of the MRI, and prevent a good image from being obtained. Modern MRI equipment are able to compensate for this distortion (artifact), improving the image quality, but this advance has its limitations. However, older spinal implants, such as older scoliosis implants, predating the 1990s transition to titanium alloy, are predominantly stainless steel, which produced even greater distortion in the MRI and a myelogram is almost always necessary.

23 What is Cervical Degenerative Disc Disease?

Degenerative disc disease (DDD) is not a clinical diagnosis in the sense that the diagnosis is made by radiologists after reviewing spinal imaging, and not on the basis of symptoms or careful examination. And since it is so common, DDD can be a problematic term, because in reality this disease is so common that it is more of a commonality among all adults— At some point in adolescence, the disc material begins to degenerate in each and all of us. This process can begin in teenagers, shown by Swischuk and coinvestigators, finding DDD on MRI in the neck and back of 26% of children under 16 years old that participated in the study. These volunteers did not have a history of any previous or current back or neck pain, or major trauma.[87]

87 *Swischuk LE, et al. Disk degenerative disease in childhood:*

At the Radiological Society of North America 2003 Scientific Assembly and Annual Meeting, further evidence was highlighted that found this process beginning in an even younger population. The MRI studies of 154 ten year-olds without a past or present history of back pain were analyzed, finding 9% of these study participants to have evidence of disc degeneration.[88] Findings such as these call into question the clinical utility of such a diagnosis. These findings also highlight one area where a more clinically useful diagnostic grading system can be developed.

The Degenerating Disc, Water Loss, and Aging

To understand the impact of disc degeneration, one must understand all of the functions of the healthy cervical disc. The disc is a cushion between each spinal segment, serving as a shock absorber, and imparts flexibility to the spine. The disc is thought to be tallest in the morning, just after waking up. Throughout the day, the cushion slowly shortens— At the end of the day after prolonged compression, from body weight alone, the disc is at its shortest, often up to approximately an inch. Supporting this is the observation by DePukey who found patients under 10 and 80 years to be on average 2% and 0.5% shorter by bedtime.[89] As the water content of the disc decreases throughout life, degeneration occurs and so the discs all shorten, and the spine becomes less flexible.

It is the water in the central component of the disc, the nucleus pulosus, that gives the center of the disc a gelatinous character, which can absorb nearly 10 times the volume of water, which is

---

Scheurermann's disease, Schmorl's nodes, and the limbu vertebra: MRI findings in 12 patients. Pediatr Radiol. 1998; 28(5):334-8.

88 *Degenerative Disc Disease: How early Does It Occur? An MRI Study of 154 Ten Year Old Children. 2003. Radiological Society of North America 2003 Scientific Assembly and Annual Meeting.*

89 *DePukey P. The physiological oscillation of the length of the body. Acta Orthop Scand 1935;6:338d*

partially lost throughout the day through mechanical pressure, similar to pressure on a wet sponge.

Spondylosis: Associated Changes in the Facet Joints and Ligaments in Relation to Disc Degeneration

Disc degeneration results in a number of other changes, all of which are described generally in a single term- spondylosis. As the disc progressively loses height by degeneration, the disc pressure increases. With less volume and increased pressure, the outer ring of the disc bulges outward from the increased pressure, causing a disc bulge. This is a very common finding. The outer ring, called the annulus fibrosus, under chronic or excessive strain, may develope fissures. These are visible on MRI. Other types of disc herniations may develop as a result. Increased abnormal motion will occur with enough degeneration which is associated with facet joint inflammation, synovial cysts, ligamentous hypertrophy, paraspinal muscle spasms, endplate inflammation and Modic Changes— all of which are features of spondylosis.

Cervical Degenerative Disc Disease: Grading on MRI

As with lumbar degenerative disc, an important issue with grading cervical degenerative disc disease is that the radiologist may not adhere to the same grading system that that next spine surgeon or radiologist might be familiar with. In one study, Jacobs and colleagues proposed a reasonable grading classification, and put this to the test, finding excellent intra-and inter-rater reliability. This 'inter-rater reliability' refers to the likelihood that different radiologists will look at the same MRI of a cervical disc degeneration and assign the same grade. The 'intra-rater reliability' refers to the likelihood that the same radiologist will assign the same cervical disc degeneration grade over and over again, were he or she to be given the same MRI or different MRI with the same features again. This is helpful to know about a classification for fairly obvious reasons. The figure below shows one proposed cervical disc degeneration grading system for MRI (Fig. 23-1). The scoring is a linear scale, from 0 to 3, in order of progressing degeneration, where the disc is normal (grade 0), darkens (grade 1), collapses and shows minimal osteophytes (grade 2), and finally develops many osteophytes (grade 3).[90]

Cervical Degenerative Disc Grading Using MRI

Figure 23-1. Cervical MRI Classification Grades: One proposed classification of increasing severity from 0 (normal) to progressing degeneration of the disc (I, top right), to early osteophyte/spur development (II, bottom left), and finally with advanced osteophyte/spur formation (III, bottom right).

---

90 *Jacobs et al. Reliable Magnetic Resonance Imaging Based on Grading System For Cervical Intervertebral Disc Degeneration. Asian Spine J. 2016; 10(1):70-74.*

Evaluating Research Showing Disc Degeneration In Pediatric Populations

It is always important when reading about research studies to not jump to any conclusions. At times, it can be difficulty to break free from the 'headline news' mentality, especialy when the article is reported via 'Headline News'. The reality is, most of the time, the conclusions that can be made from scientific studies in medicine are incredibly limited. In order to conduct a good research study, a vary narrow question is asked. The design of the study serves to answer that question specifically. The answer will be incredibly narrow as well, meaning that it cannot be broadly applicable. For example, returning to the previous study example, wherein almost 10% of 10 year olds had cervical and/or lumbar disc degeneration. In fact, it is not true to say that 10% of all 10 year olds have disc degeneration because it is not known if the volunteers have much in common with the characteristics of a general population. One analogy that most are familiar with is bias that results from polling. Among other things, polls don't include the input of people that hate answering polls, author included— therefore, the results of polls most consider that biasto say the very least.

Now, consider another study designed to determine the frequency of disc degeneration in pediatric patients with symptoms of back or neck pain. In order to limit bias, a hypothesis is made before the study is designed and conducted. However, after two years of collecting data, instead of spending more money to collect data for each small question, suppose the data was 'mined'. But the issue is that data is a form of bias. If one now knows that there are clusters of unusual and exciting results, hypotheses are created to explain the results and this data is examined (a post-hoc analysis). Exciting results from post-hoc analyses are heavily biased. For more digression into the difference between the two, one editorial by Helmut Schuhlen in the *European Heart Journal* explains the application of this concept to a real world trial for the treatment of myocardial infarction.[91]

Cervical Disc Degeneration

Cervical disc degeneration is considered a diagnosis, which creates confusion for patients. Having neck pain and an MRI finding of cervical disc degeneration is not necessarily evidence of a cause and effect relationship. The diagnostic process may involve additional testing, visiting a spinal specialist, and determining which types of treatments relieve certain symptoms. For example, it is often argued that cervical muscle spasms are the more common cause of neck pain. Therefore, an intramuscular injection with steroids may be more effective.

Often, the lines are blurred between a disease and a natural process of aging. Is male pattern baldness a disease at age 60? There is no defined threshold between a disease and a naturally occurring finding. For example, if 20, 30, and 50% of the population have a finding at ages 30, 40, and 60, is it a pathology? A disease is generally defined as, " 1. a disordered or incorrectly functioning organ, part, structure, or system...[92] There are many varying definitions but most agree in that a disease is due to disordered or abnormally functioning anatomy. Another way to look at this is that unless one is an immortal, common manifestations of aging are inherent and not a sign of a 'disordered or incorrectly functioning' organ, part, structure, or system.

---

91 *Schuhlen H. Pre-specified vs. post-hoc subgroup analyses: are we weiser before or after a trial has been performed? European Heart Journal 35(31):2055-2057: 2014.*

92 *"http://www.dictionary.com, accessed January 1,2019"*

Inflammatory Endplate Changes

The diagnostic workup and clinical history are arguably the most helpful in determining the underlying causes of neck pain. However, one feature associated with cervical DDD are inflammatory changes adjacent to the disc, in the bone of the vertebrae above and below. The content of water decreases in the disc as one ages. The disc loses volume and eventually loses height. Inflammation can set in at the junctions of the disc and bone above and below, causing inflammatory changes in the endplate. Inflammatory changes in the endplate are commonly referred to as Modic Changes, and have an early inflammatory component, called Type I Modic Changes. These are followed by changes of chronic inflammation, which are replaced by less inflammation, and chronic changes such as thicking of density of the endplates (sclerosis), and decreased vascularity, which is Type II Modic Changes. These distinctions are identified on MRI (Fig. 23-2).

Modic Changes

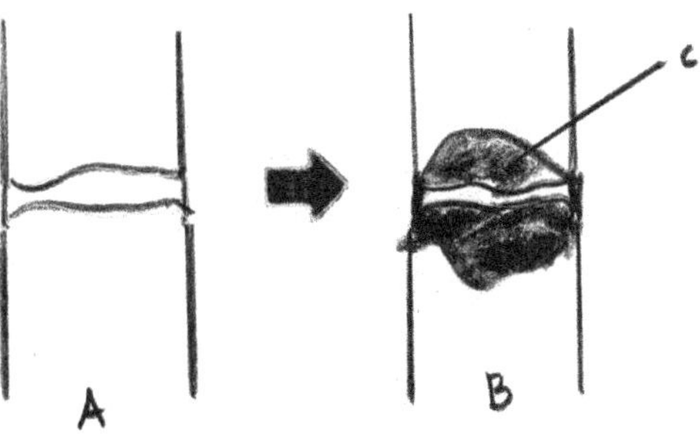

Figure 23-2. Modic changes (very simplified diagram) are inflammatory changes in the normal endplates(A) result in Type I changes of marrow inflammation and edema (c) and evntually sclerosis of the vessels and chronic

changes of type II seen in the endplates (B). Type III changes are occasionally described, which are a very advanced stage of extensive calcification of the endplates (not shown). The classification system is based on T1 and T2 MRI characteristics.

The Utilization of Research Data In Advertising

Before continuing with the topic of disc degeneration, it is important to review a few general advertising practices in the treatment of disc degeneration or related symptoms that the author has come across when reading about new products. After all, disc degeneration is present in all of us. With the many products in competition with each other, advertisements often emphasize results of research studies— as this adds an element of legitimacy. As the astute reader knows, research has many different levels of quality.

First, the research results can either be published in a journal or it can be an internal study conducted by the manufacturer, or conducted in the loosest description of the word. A study published in a journal has the advantages that it was submitted to journal reviewers, who are gatekeepers to the journal. Today, with the growing number of medical journals, some journals are much more selective than others. Journal selectiveness usually correlates to it's impact factor (IF), a numerical score. Typically, better quality studies are published in journals that have a higher IF and hence a greater likelihood that readers will encounter the study. If there is no available reference to the research advertising claim (similar to the footnote below), then the advertising claim should be shrewdly ignored.

Not all patients are comfortable, or have the time to research advertising claims and educate themselves on the necessary subjects to make an informed decision. It is an undertaking, and unless someone is an expert in that relevant healthcare subject and completely understands the research study in question, and also, medical statistics, consider discussing the product/treatment with your healthcare provider. After all, the existence of research in advertising is carefully organized to convince the potential customer to commit to buying the product. Therefore, asking clarifiying questions to the party trying to sell the product can be less helpful.

One trend is the reliance of advertisers on percentages in advertising. Simply put, the higher the percentage, the more of a potential impact this advertising will make. Hypothetically, one example has the description, "99% improvement in satisfaction" printed on the label. This is basically a guarantee— nearly everyone is satisfied, and therefore it is effective. After the initial excitement, hopefully prior to buying the product, the shrewd patient must take over and begin to assess these claims. First, the above statement is intentionally very vague. Most retailers will not know all the details, and this is because they are rarely asked. Also, just like the advertising, the claims made by the seller should be reviewed as well. Overall, this can become a monumental task.

The more one understands how studies are conducted and research, either of two things might happen. Advertising claims such as the aforementioned example lose appeal and are disregarded outright— Alternatively, more questions arise. Returning to the product with '99% improvement in satisfaction', it was determined from the same study that a 10 point scale of increasing satisfaction was used, from 1 to 10. It turns out that this study evaluated a small group of the research patients (in a post-hoc subgroup analysis). In this group, with a starting score of 1.0, the score improved from 1.0 to 1.99 out of a possible 10, which is a small improvement, but technically a 99% increase.

Also, upon further review of the hypothetical study, the satisfaction scoring system was one that the reader was familiar with and it was noted that the scoring system uses a well-known questionnaire, and an improvement of atleast 2 points is needed for the patient to recognize a minimum clinically important difference (MCID). Not all scales have an MCID, but it is pragmatic to know this in advance when evaluating grading tools for studies that examine small improvements in satisfaction. Overall, the improvement of 0.9 did not exceed the 2 points needed for MCID and therefore if the starting satisfaction were 1.0, a noticeable improvement may not be achieved. However, there is still too little known about the study to make many other statements. The example was created to emphasize how even the most dismal results can be utilized in a way to sell a product.

Advertising of Dissimilar Treatments Using Research From The Same Study- Unsubstantiated Conclusions

Moreover, it never ceases to amaze the author how even completely unrelated research can be used in an advertisement to the same effect. Let's say in one advertisement regarding neck pain the reader evaluates the claims that, "chiropractic (spinal manipulation) is very helpful for pediatric patients, as one recent study demonstrated that disc degeneration can be present in 9% of 10 year-olds." Again, little is known about the treatment, and less is known about the research. It turns out that the research that was quoted was of *volunteers without back pain* and since this study did not evaluate chiropractic, and it most certainly did not evaluate chiropractic in minors without symptoms, the two statements are unequivocally unrelated. The deception that lies in the hypothetical example above are in fact two unqualified statements— that disc degeneration must cause symptoms (false), and it must be implied that chiropractic must be a valid treatment for neck pain when established that the pain is caused by disc degeneration. Anecdotally drawing a link between disc degneration and neck pain is very difficult. Since there is no proven way to reverse disc degeneration, any treatments that might be perceived as successful, could just as well be treating an unidentified process. Recall again, that disc degeneration does not always cause pain. This last example is equally misleading because the reader is dragged through several assumptions, as if these were common knowledge, in order to reach a favorable conclusion.

In summary, it can be challenging without prior experience in in healthcare or a related field to assess healthcare products and find claims that are substantiated. Not only that, one must be confident in their own findings if they expect to use this for a personal healthcare decision. If at any time the reader is in doubt, it is just as reasonable and recommended to develop a plan with a trusted healthcare provider that will bring years of experience and additional considerations to help make the best joint decision with his or her patient.

24 What is a Cervical Disc Herniation?

The cervical intervertebral disc is a shock absorber located between each segment of bone throughout the spine. Segments, called vertebral bodies, or vertebra, provide the foundation and structure that allows us to be upright. The disc material is contained within the disc space by a tough, fibrous ring called the annulus fibrosus. The disc material in the center is gelatinous, made up mostly of water and proteoglycans (amino acids) termed the nucleus pulposus. Over time, the entire disc will lose integrity, much like a tire on a car. The outer ring of the disc, the annulus, can form a defect where disc material can extrude into the spinal canal.

There are many ways that a disc can herniate into the spinal canal. Disc herniations are among the most common causes of back and leg pain (Fig. 24-1). It is also very common to find multiple disc herniations on an MRI at several different levels, and this does not necessarily correlate with the severity of a back condition.

This is because disc herniations may or may not be contributing to your symptoms. In fact, as we read earlier in the introduction section, disc herniations can be observed on MRI in upwards of 50-60% of asymptomatic volunteers in their thirties!

Disc Herniations Can Cause Pain By Compression of Neighboring Nerve Root(s)

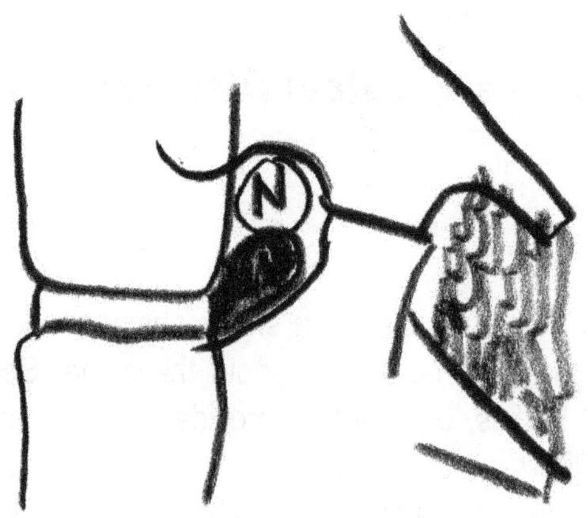

Figure 24-1. A herniated cervical disc (black, adjacent to 'N') can put pressure on one or several nerves in close proximity, especially the exiting cervical nerve root (N) as it courses near the disc space while exiting the neural foramen. Nerve compression causes pain, complaints of sensory symptoms in the same region, occasionally a burning feeling, and even weakness.

25 What Are the Different Types of Cervical Disc Herniations?

A cervical disc herniation goes by many names. Most of the differences are radiographic classifcations only, and while some forms are more frequently associated with certain neurologic symptoms than others, independtly, the various forms that a cervical disc herniation can take does not impact the clinical management, but some types or more likely to be associated with symptoms than others.

Cervical Disc Herniations: 'Contained' or 'Not Contained' By The Annulus

Cervical disc herniations appear in many forms. The most common is a very slight increase in the diameter of the whole disc space due to collapse of the disc space, called a disc bulge (Fig 25-1). The easiest way to characterize most other disc herniations are as contained (Fig. 25-2) or non-contained disc herniations (Fig. 25-3). This refers to whether or not the annulus fibrosus, the outer ring of the disc is intact or not. A disc protrusion was at one point referring to a disc herniation where the nucleus pulposis, or disc material, is contained within the annulus. More commonly, a protrusion refers to a relatively narrow transverse width of the disc when compared to that of the disc it is arising from. Another way that disc protrusions can be distinguished from disc bulges is that one classification subdivides the annulus by 360 degrees (despite not being a perfect circle). If the disc material projects beyond the vertebral body, but across less than than 90 degrees of the ring, then this meets the criteria for a protrusion.

The Disc Bulge: A Manifestation of Degeneration and Pressure In The Disc Space

A disc bulge is where disc material projects beyond the margin of the vertebral body over more than 1/4 of the circumference. This is more commonly a clinical problem in the lumbosacral spine than with the cervical spine as the lumbar disc is under greater pressure resulting from the weight of the upper extremities, chest, and abdomen. Another way of conceptualizing disc bulging is that disc degenerates, loses height, and the annulus, being the same surface area, will bulge outward (figure). This also occurs with the ligaments surrounding the collapses disc. base of the disc is equal to, or greater than half the disc diameter (example b in the diagram). These are the most common and occur in patients with and without symptoms. These frequently can cause symptoms on both sides, due to how concentric they are.

The Disc Bulge

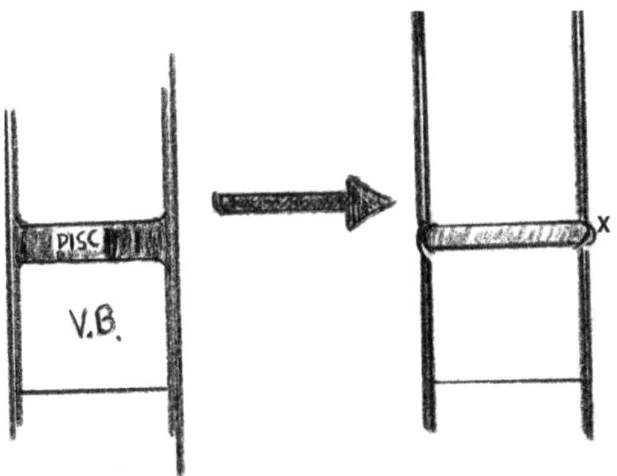

Figure 25-1. Disc Bulging is concentric, and occurs when the height of the disc space decreases due to degeneration, but the height of the adjacent anterior and posterior longitudinal ligaments and annulus do not lose height. Instead, they bulge, which is analgous to wearing the wrong size scrub pants— because somone felt that 5XL and 5XS was uncertain of the Bell Curve and ordered equal proportions as if there were equal demand to medium. On most people below 7 feet tall, the 5 XL gives the pant leg an appearance like an accordian. This excess that is bunched up is like the anterior longitudinal ligament, which contributes to stenosis.

Cervical Disc Protrusion

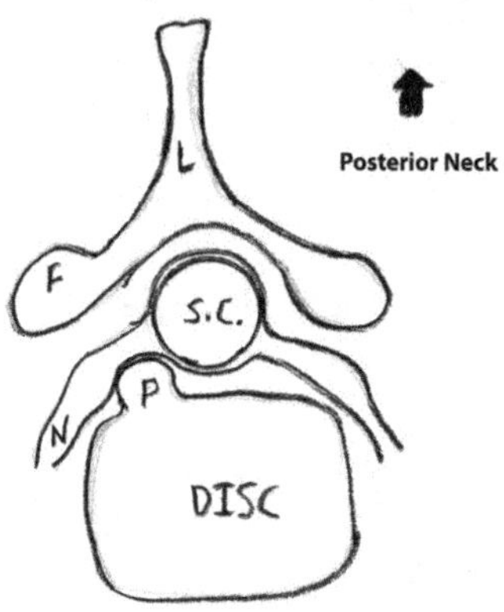

Figure 25-2. Cervical disc protrusion: Cross section of the cervical spine is shown, with the back of the neck in the direction of the arrow. The herniated disc material, the protrusion (P), is compressing the nerve (N) as it exits the spinal cord (S.C.). Larger disc herniations can compress the nerve in the foramen between the disc and facet (F). When the disc material is contained within the annulus and with a narrow width relative to the parent disc, it is called a protrusion. L- lamina.

Extrusion- Disc Material Outside Of The Annulus

Disc herniations that are outside of the annulus are most likely to cause symptoms for two reasons. They are more likely to compress nerve roots, and also because the disc material from the nucleus pulposus is very inflammatory, and the nerve root is sensative to the 'chemicals' in the disc space. In an extrusion, disc material has passed through a defect in the disc wall, and is in continuity with the disc space, and also more frequently has a base relatively more narrow than the dome. The disc extrusions usually exit through a small annular tear, which is most often a vertical tear, as the fibers are vertically oriented. Most often, extrusions cause symptoms, presumably as inflammatory material from the nucleus residing outside of the disc space to inflame an exiting spinal root.

Cervical Disc Extrusion (or 'Prolapse')

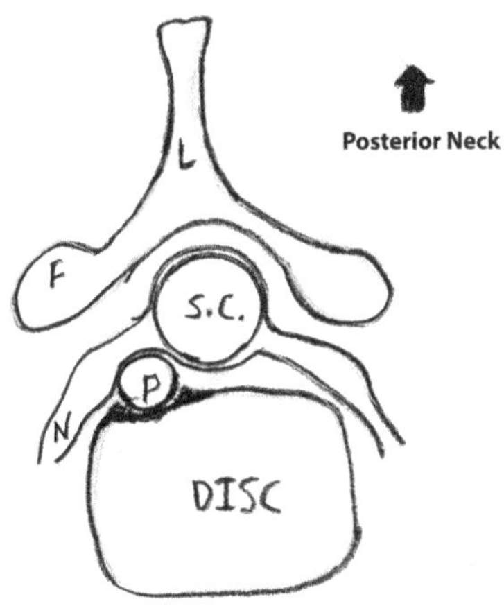

Figure 25-3. Cervical disc extrusion (prolapse): same orientation and labelling as in preceding figure. Disc material (P) is no longer contained within the annulus, having exited through an annular fissure. This example above is of a cervical disc extrusion, which is defined as a disc fragment outside of the annulus, but contiguous with the disc space. Therefore, the final example of a noncontained disc herniation is a sequestration, where the material is noncontiguous with the disc space.

Sequestration- Outside of the Annulus and Not Adjacent To the Disc Space

Last, the disc sequestration is a term for disc extrusions that are found away from the disc space, and not in direct continuity with the disc space. This means that the space in between the disc and the disc space has been filled usually with the dura returning to its original position. Occasionally, the discs will have been referred to as 'migrated', as in the example in the figure below, of a C5-6 disc sequestration, where the disc fragment has left the C5-6 disc space and migrated behind the vertebral body of C6 (Fig. 25-4). Migrated discs can still return to the disc space— generically termed 'regression', when seen on an MRI report.[93] Usually this herniation is not so far that it is difficult to tell what disc this material arose from, especially in the cervical spine. Disc material is located away from the disc space, not in continuity. This is the least commonly seen and most often when they are encountered, they are associated with symptoms.

---

93 *Turk O and Yaldiz C. Spontaneous regression of cervical discs: Retrospective analysis of 14 cases. Medicine. 98(7):2019.*

Cervical Disc Sequestration

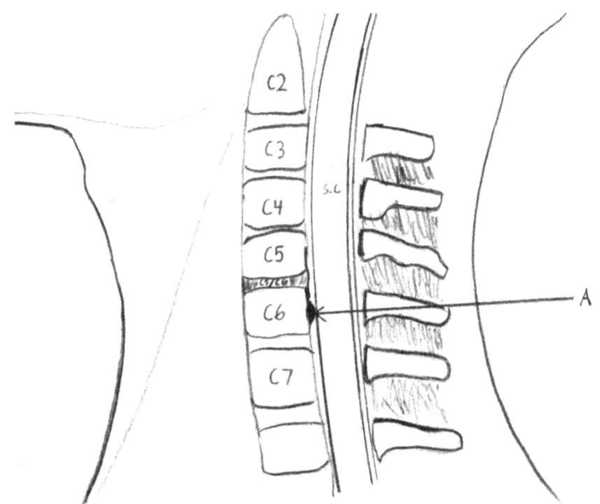

Figure 25-4. Cervical Disc Sequestration, sagittal cross section of the neck, demonstrating degeneration of the C5-6 disc space, with migration of the disc downward (caudally) with the position behind (posterior) the C6 vertebral body (A).

Summary

There are many terms that all refer to types of cervical disc herniations. Due to the varied experience and background of the many radiologists, these numerous terms— bulge, protrusion, extrusion, herniation, prolapse, and sequestration— all describe a similar process of a disc herniation. These distinctions are largely academic. Studying these distinctions are less important than understanding their impact on the local anatomy, meaning, what structures are being compressed, and what degree of stenosis has resulted, if any. These terms have been thought to represent a spectrum of increased symptom severity— Meaning, as the disc leaves the disc space (extrusion), and even migrates (sequestered), an increasing likelihood of neurologic deficit or intractable pain can be encountered (Fig. 25-5). It is also important to recognize that the classification of the disc herniation is arbitary and does not change the management on the basis of classification, but on a variety of factors such as the presence of neurologic deficits, signs, symptoms, and failure to respond with non-surgical measures.

Cervical Disc Herniations

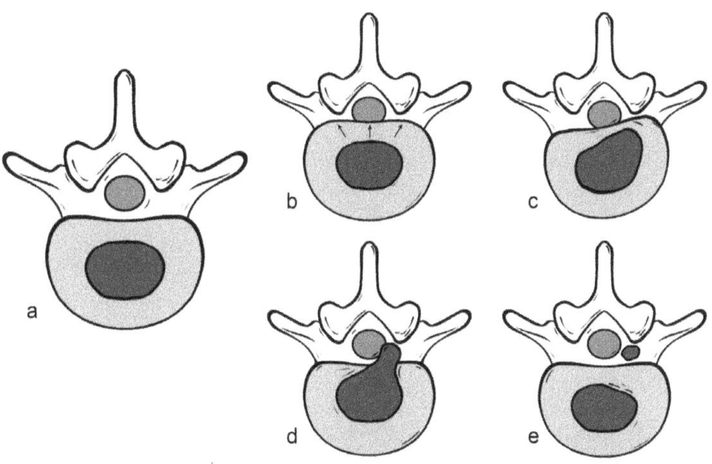

Figure 25-5. Diagram depicting the various types of disc hernations.[94] *Image A shows the normal cross section of the disc space, with a large ring surrounding the darker center. B. A disc bulge is a broad projection of the disc evenly outside of the disc space and is seen with disc space collapse. C. A protrusion is where a small portion of the disc projects outside of the disc space, with a contained annulus and is less than 90 degrees width, if the disc is divided into four quadrants of 90 degrees (although the true shape is ovoid. D. A disc extrusion occurs when a fragment exits the annulus, but is in continuity with the disc space. E. A sequestration may occur when the disc fragment is no longer in continuity with the disc.*

94 *From The Low Back Pain Guide, with permission.*

26 What is Cervical Stenosis?

In the context of medicine, stenosis is a term that implies an abnormal degree of narrowing of any natural channel from one cavity to another in the body. There are varying degrees of stenosis directly as a result of cervical disc degeneration, making this diagnosis almost as common as disc degeneration. Just the same with disc degeneration (see chapter 22, disc degeneration), in most people, there are multiple levels that have stenosis, making it difficult to identify specific instances where stenosis may be causing symptoms. Typically, milder degrees of stenosis do not cause nerve compression, and are unlikely a cause of pain. Therefore, most cases of both disc degeneration and stenosis are incidental findings and do not need treatment.

Stenosis: Initial Radiographic Assessment

At any spinal level, there are two locations where stenosis can occur, the central canal and neural formaen. Radiologists will comment on the presence or absence of stenosis at each level of your cervical spine and the location. Next, they will comment on the degree of stenosis, when present. The central canal is the larger of the two, is posterior to the disc, and contains the spinal cord (Fig 26-1).

Understanding Sagittal and Axial-Oriented Spinal Imaging

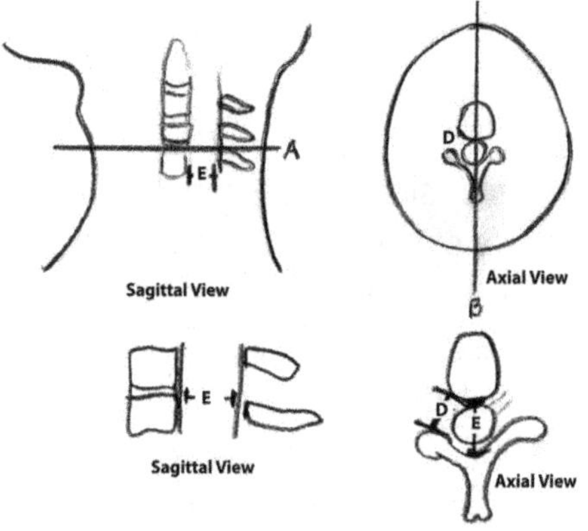

Figure 26-1. Sagittal and axial oriented (simplified diagram) views forms the basis of understanding imaging of three-dimensional space (of the spine). A sagittal view in the top left image shows a vertical cross section of the spine in relation to the head and neck. The middle of the central canal is labeled E. The cross section of line 'A' is represented in axial imaging in the top right image, where the cross section 'B' again represents in turn the line 'A' from the top left sagittal image. The enlarged spinal segments from each image are shown just below in the same figure to illustrate how the central canal (E) and neuro foramen (D) are represented. From understanding

these types of representations (projections), it becomes clear why the neural foramen is not visible on the sagittal view in this example as the middle of the body does not contain the right or left neural foramina, which are approximately one centimeter to the left or right of the midline.

The spinal cord is contained in the central canal and is filled with cerebrospinal fluid which is contained by the dura (Fig. 26-2). Stenosis of the central canal can then be described as central, or paracentral and either can cause nerve or spinal cord compression. At each level of the cervical spine, a pair of nerves exit the neural foramen. As mentioned, the spinal cord is comprised of nerves that run to and from the brain and is in the central canal of the spine. The nerves exit to the right and the left through a neural foramen. Neural foraminal stenosis is narrowing of the channel where the nerve courses through the spine.

Increased Chances of Symptoms With Greater Degrees of Stenosis

Eventually, disc degeneration occurs and then the disc will begin to slowly shorten (collapse has a connotation of complete loss of height, but is often used for any degree of shortening of the disc space), which in turn causes buckling of the annulus fibrosus. The annulus fibrosus is a tough ring surrounding the the disc space. Other stabilizing ligaments support the disc in front of and behind of the cervical spine and maintain alignment.

Determining what degree of stenosis is significant is difficult without medical training and requires an understanding various elements of the clinical picture. First, the degree of stenosis is certainly very important, especially in the presence of nerve or spinal cord compression. Also, the presence or absence of painful complaints, especially pain radiating down the arm, is often a hallmark of cervical radiculopathy, or clinical nerve root compression, but this arm pain is not always related to cervical radiculopathy.[95]

Stenosis is occasionally graded as 'mild', 'moderate', and 'severe' and these qualitative terms differ (Fig. 25-3). Just exactly what the variation 'moderately severe' means to the patient and what the clinical relevance is, remains to be seen. Qualitative grading of stenosis for a particular study may vary in interpretation, which is a common hurdle with some grading scales.

Central Canal and Neural Foramen

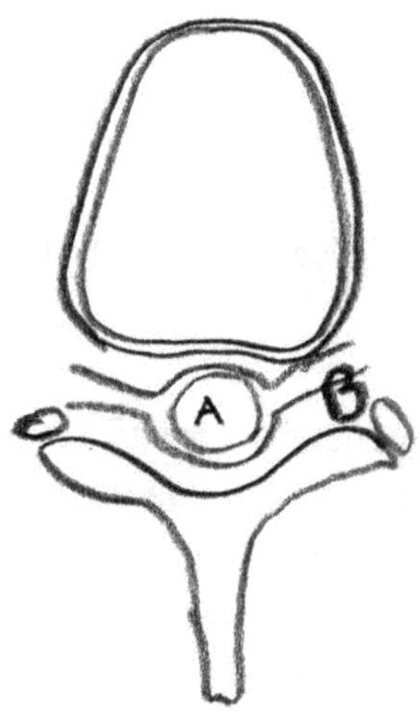

Figure 26-2. Cervical Spine, Illustration depicting transverse cross section across the level of a cervical disc. Posterior to the disc, the central canal is located, labelled A. The spinal cord is a larger bundle of nerve tissue, and at each level, a pair of nerve exit on the right and left side through the neu-

---

95 *Pain Radiating Down The Extremity has numerous causes including advanced osteoarthritis, nerve entrapment outside of the spine, and even in the case of the left arm can be a sign of cardiac disease. See Cervical Radiculopathy, and also Cervical Red Flag Signs.*

ral foramen, labelled B. The foramen is bordered by the disc, vertebral body, bony pedicle above, and the facet joint.

The Various Grades Of Cervical Foraminal Stenosis

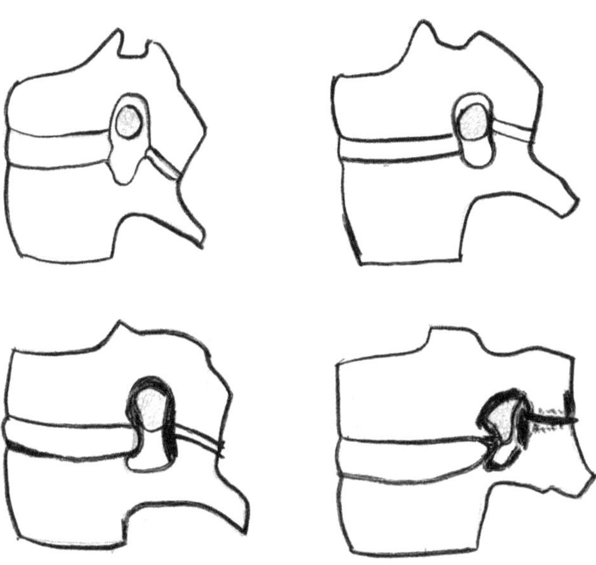

Figure 26-3. Cervical Foraminal Stenosis: One grading proposal by There are various grades of cervical foraminal stenosis. Proposals may require specific types of MRI reconstructions such as sagittal[96] or axial[97]. In general, the scales are progressive, beginning with the absence of stenosis (top left), early contact with the nerve, but without any compression (which would be defined as decreasing cross-sectional area; top right), compression with less than 50% reduction of the nerve area (bottom left), and severe stenosis resulting in greater than 50% compression(bottom right).

---

96 *Park HJ, et al. A practical MRI grading system for cervical foraminal stenosis based on oblique sagittal images. Br J Radiol 2013; 86.*

97 *Kim S, et al. A New MRI Grading System for Cervical Foraminal Stenosis Based on Axial T2-Weighted Images. Korean J Radiol 2015; 16(6):1294-1302.*

27 Do I Need Contrast 'Dye' With My Imaging?

Medical imaging has transformed over the past 100 years, which was approximately the duration of time since the widespread acceptance of x-rays as a medical imaging procedure in the United States. One early x-ray or CT drawback is the inability to visualize soft tissue structures directly or indirectly. This gave rise to the use of contrast agents, such as iodine-based or barium-sulfate. Contrast agents work differently and depend on several factors: the specific contrast agent itself and it's unique chemical properties, it's interaction with ionizing radiation (or in a magnetic field in the case of an MRI), the route of administration (for the spine, intravenous or intrathecal)[98], and at what time the imaging is obtained.

98 *A CT myelogram uses intrathecal contrast— for more information, see the section on CT imaging.*

Contrasted CT scans

Contrast in a CT scan of the spine is not frequently used, and an MRI is more helpful, with or without contrast. In a contrasted CT scan, known diseases and for spinal imaging, this refers to intravenous contrast, which is given as an injection in the veins just prior to the start of the imaging study. Soft tissue anatomy in the central nervous system does not appear more clearly with a CT with contrast, as the blood-brain barrier, as special barrier protecting the central nervous system, does not allow for larger molecules such as iodinated contrast to enter the healthy brain. Moreover, iodinated contrast is thought to be neurotoxic.[99]

Contrasted MRI Scans

For CT studies, iodinated contrast is used, and for MRI studies, gadolinium-based contrast agents (GBCAs) are used. The principles are the same, with the goal to raise the likelihood of detection of certain anatomy. The only other route that contrast is given in a spinal study is the CT myelogram, which is delivered by a spinal injection into the cerebrospinal fluid, which will be discussed in a separate section.

The authors experience echoes that of many other clinicians that a CT with intravenous contrast is not very useful in diagnosis and treatment planning. In fact, in practice, this author has rarely encountered a spinal surgeon who incorporates a contrasted CT scan into the general spine practice.

Gadolinium is a paramagnetic chemical, which means that it weakly attracts to a magnet but does not have permanent magnetic

---

99 *Junck L and Marshall WH. Neurotoxicity of radiological contrast agents. Ann Neurol. 13(5):469-84, 1983.*

properties, which makes it useful in some instances to change the appearance of tissues an MRI. It was noted that gadolinium can 'enhance' the appearance of certain pathologies that have increased perfusion, as one would expect that some (but not all) tumors, inflammation, and acute injuries would have increased blood flow, allowing the gadolinium to reach the tissues of interest in greater quantity. Gadolinium has been in use for more than 30 years.[100]

Adverse Effects Associated With Gadolinium

Risks of gadolinium range from mild to life-threatening, with some risks that scientists are still trying to understand the long term implications. Similar to iodinated contrast, gadolinium also carries common risks such as worsening renal impairment in patients with chronic kidney disease, as well as hypersensitivity reactions. Up to 5% of patients may report a headache after gadolinium administration. However, with any medication, a whole host of side effects are reported by patients, and as a result, the complete list of reported symptoms and any safety reports can bee found on FDA.gov, which is frequently updated.

One other concern with GBCAs use is that it will impair the visualization of lesions that are visible without contrast. Gadolinium is a paramagetic molecule, which has a distinctly different MRI appearance (GBCAs appear bright on T1 MRI sequences). However, relatively few tissues are naturally bright-appearing on T1 MRI sequences. This requires a careful comparison of T1 MRI sequences before contrast is administered, called a noncontrast

---

100 *Bassett M. Thirty years later, questions remain on gadolinium-based contrast agent retention. In Radiological Society of North America. Source: https://www.rsna.org/news/2019/April/Gadolinium-Based-Contrast-Agent-Retention*

sequence. This is the rationale for an MRI test ordered both 'with and without contrast'.

As a result, if further MRI testing is required, contrast will remain in the system for a variable duration, preventing the use of noncontrast MRI. Using one specific example, gadopentetate dimeglumine(trade name: Magnevist), one type of GBCAs that you may receive, shows 91% clearance after 24 hours through the urine (see FDA data link below). For the most part, diseases with increased blood vessel formation or tissues with relatively greater perfusion will appear brighter after administration of gadolinium, increasing the chances that said diseases are diagnosed. Examples include some neoplasms, areas of inflammation, and even scar tissue can appear clearly after contrast is administered.

Nephrogenic Systemic Fibrosis (NSF)

Nephrogenic Systemic Fibrosis (NSF) is a rare complication of GBCA use in patients with kidney impairment. GBCAs are cleared by the kidneys. In patients with kidney impairment and who had previously received GBCAs, reports of a system wide fibrosis affecting the skin, muscle, and internal organs have been documented. It is thought that elevated gadolinium dosing or repeat dosing serves as a risk.[101] If you have chronic kidney disease, there is still a risk of renal failure with GBCA use apart from the less common development of NSF.

---

101 *FDA safety, dosing, precautions and other cautionary reports of gadopenatate dimeglumine is reported in: https://www.accessdata.fda.gov/drugsatfda_docs/label/2018/019596s063lbl.pdf*

Contrasted Spinal MRI Studies Are Not Routinely Used For Most Spinal Degenerative Diseases

Contrast is only helpful in specific disease processes, and most often, is not helpful for routine diagnostic imaging. The majority of clinical problems are degenerative spinal disorders and MRI imaging with contrast is not required for acute onset neck and arm pain. Also, these substances can be associated with severe allergic reactions and kidney failure among other conditions. For that reason, the risks outweighs the potential benefits of administering contrast during every imaging study.

Gadolinium Deposition Disease

In 2015, the FDA released a report commenting on recent studies that found that patients that had more than four contrasted MRIs were found to have brain deposits of gadolinium, particularly in the dentate nucleus and globus pallidum in the brain.[102] It was later realized that these deposits were not confined to the brain, and although it was not identified if these findings were harmful, and GBCA use was not restricted or limited at that time.[103] To date, the inclusion of the recognition of gadolinium deposition as a risk of GBCA administration also includes the knowledge that their is no associated symptoms linked to this deposition. However, very rarely, reports of fatigue and other vague complaints have published, which will be very difficult to link to gadolinium deposition as

102 *https://www.fda.gov/drugs/drug-safety-and-availability/fda-drug-safety-communication-fda-evaluating-risk-brain-deposits-repeated-use-gadolinium-based*

103 *https://www.fda.gov/drugs/drug-safety-and-availability/fda-drug-safety-communication-fda-identifies-no-harmful-effects-date-brain-retention-gadolinium*

it is very nonspecific.[104]

Exploration of the Potential Relationship Between MRI Use and DNA Damage

In 2015, researchers began probing the possibility if there was a relationship between MRI use and DNA damage. A review heretofor found several interesting studies, none of which were designed to identify MRI with or without GBCA as a risk for DNA damage.[105] Genetics and cancer is a very complex topic, and one focus of research in determing if MRI and GBCAs are carcinogenic (a cancer risk) is through the demonstration of DNA damage and with either increased or decreased functioning of the inherent DNA repair mechanims. Ionizing radiation can damage DNA, which is the radiation required for X-rays and CT Scans.[106] Gadolinium-enhanced cardiac MRI has been studied more recently in 2018, which did find increases in DNA repair markers, but when evaluating other molecules typically seen in the presence of DNA damage, there was no significant change.[107] Ultimately, as with other recently identified findngs such as with gadolinium deposition, there is insufficient evidence to draw any conclusions as to the significance of these observations at this time.

---

104 *FDA update on Gadolinium. https://www.fda.gov/media/116492/download*

105 *Vijayalaxmi K et al, Magnetic resonance imaging (MRI): a review of genetic damage investigations. Mutation Research/Reviews in Mutation Research. 2015 764:51-63.*

106 *Hill MA. Comments on potential health effects of MRI-induced DNA lesions: quality is more important to consider than quantity. Eur Heart J Cardiovasc Imaging. 2016 17(11):1230-1238.*

107 *McDonald JS et al. Gadolinium-enhanced cardiac MR exams of human subjects are associated with significant increases in the DNA repair marker 53BP1, but not the damage marker γH2AX. PLoS One. 2018; 13(1).*

Summary

The decision to use a gadolinium-based contrast agent is carefully considered by your physician or provider. As such, the workup and clinical care for a spinal degenerative condition is patient-specific, and in order to obtain a complete understanding of your need for a contrasted MRI, it will come from having an open dialogue with your physician or provider. GBCAs are associated some adverse risks, some of which have an indeterminate significance at this time. For an up to date reference on the use of Contrast, a comprehensive manual is frequently updated and available as a free download from the The American College of Radiology (ACR) website.[108]

---

108 *See https://www.acr.org/Clinical-Resources/Contrast-Manual . This manual is produced by the ACR 'Committee on Drugs and Contrast Media' comprised of leaders in the radiology field, and incorporates new information, atleast on an annual basis by the ACR. In the interest of informed consent, it is comendable that this material is free to download by all. However, the volume and complexity of information contained in manuals like these may serve as a insurmountable obstacle to a self-directed education on the topic and a hindrance to informed consent.*

28 What is Cervical Subluxation?

Cervical subluxation is the shift in position horizontally (anterior or posterior translation), of one cervical vertebra across the level below (Fig 28-1). Subluxation is analgous to spondylolisthesis, which is almost exclusively used regarding the lumbar spine. is also known as the “slip” in the spine. The most common cause of this condition is a result of degenerative disc disease (DDD). After the disc degenerates to the point of losing substantial height, the fibrous ligaments and the touch annulus that surrounds the disc space does not lose height. No longer under tension, the ligaments and annulus buckle, and at the level of the disc, is now free to move anteriorly or posteriorly.

Subluxation

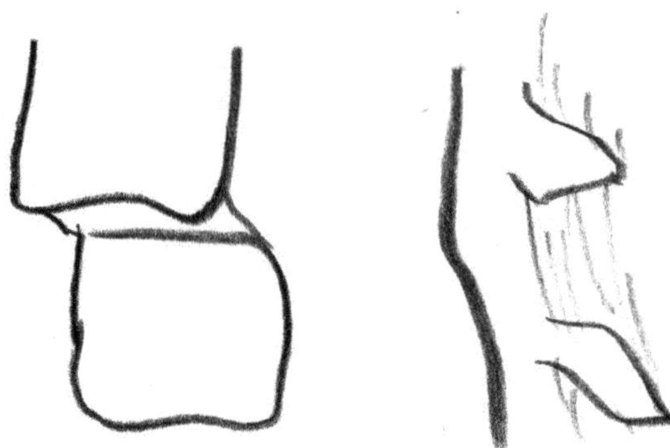

Figure 28-1. Cervical subluxation. The prevailing hypothesis of cervical disc degeneration is that disc degeneration and collapse results in ligamentous laxity, and then horizontal motion of one cervical vertebra over the other.

Degenerative Disease Creates Conditions For SubluxationTo Occur

Cervical degenerative disease eventually results in the loss of disc volume, as mostly water loss occurs and eventually the cushioning that separates the two endplates of the vertebral bodies starts to decrease in thickiness, which is referred to as a loss of disc height. The suspensory ligaments in front and behind of the disc space that are usually taut (Fig. 28-2). However, anterior and posterior longitudinal ligaments, and interspinous ligaments will relax and buckle, no longer being under maximal stretch, creating laxity and some degree of instability (Fig 28-2, 'B'). The supporting forces that hold two levels together are gone and an abnormal sliding motion can occur horizontally at the disc level between the two vertebral bodies ('C' in Fig. 28-2).

Cervical Disc Degeneration As a Precursor To Subluxation

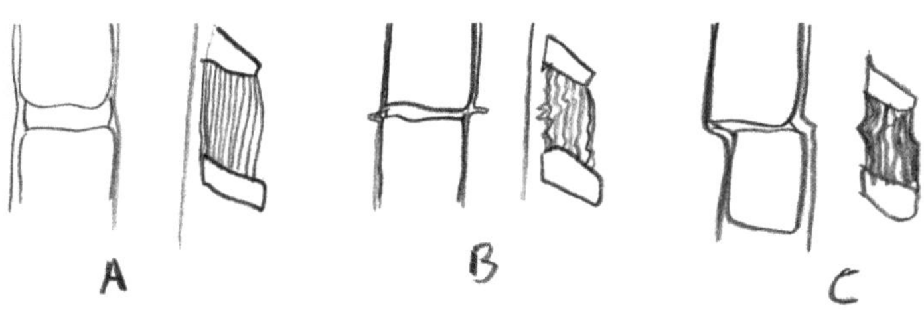

Figure 28-2. Cervical Disc Degeneration Results In a Gradual Change in Disc Height (A, left, with normal ligament tension and disc height), resulting in buckling of the ligaments (B, center), and eventually the laxity of the cervical spinal ligaments allows for the upper vertebra to translate forward or backwards (C, left).

Cervical Kyphosis

Shortening of the cervical discs leads to a shortening of the anterior aspect of the cervical spine, but without change in length of the posterior 'column' of the cervical region. When this happens, the neck starts to 'tip' forward, an alignment called cervical kyphosis (Fig. 28-3). Eventually, kyphosis can lead to significant narrowing of the neural foramen and central canal (Fig. 28-4). Kyphosis places patients at greater risk for neck pain, subluxation, disc herniation, and overall a decreased quality of life.

Degeneration of the Cervical Disc Reverses The Normal Lordotic Posture Of The Neck

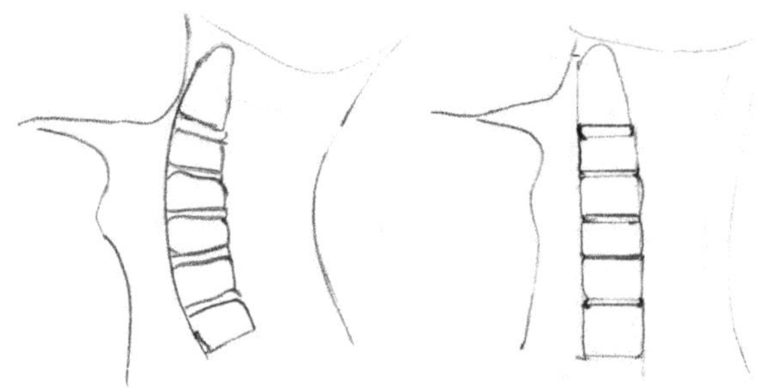

Segmental Kyphotic Changes At The Disc Level

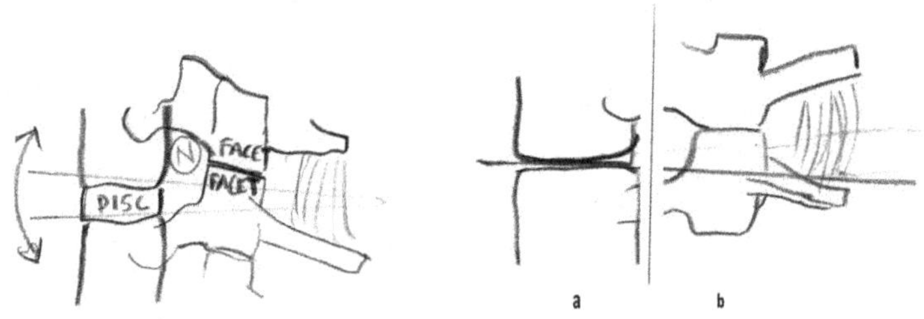

Figure 28-3. Cervical Kyphosis. The process of shortening of the cervical disc results in a straightening of the neck, as seen in the figure above (top). When a radiologist describes the overall cervical alignment on imaging and observes straightening of the cervical levels, but not to the degree that results in 'regional' kyphosis, as seen in the normal thoracic spinal alignment, this may be referred to as 'reversal of the cervical lordosis'. Sometimes when a single level is collapsed and the angle of a single disc space is kyphotic this can be referred to as segmental kyphosis (Figure below). Notice in the below

figure that disc collapse shortens the anterior 'column' (left of the line, marked a), while the posterior 'column' remains the same length (right of the line, marked b).

Kyphosis May Occur Before Disc Degeneration, Which Can Alleviate Painful Nerve Compression

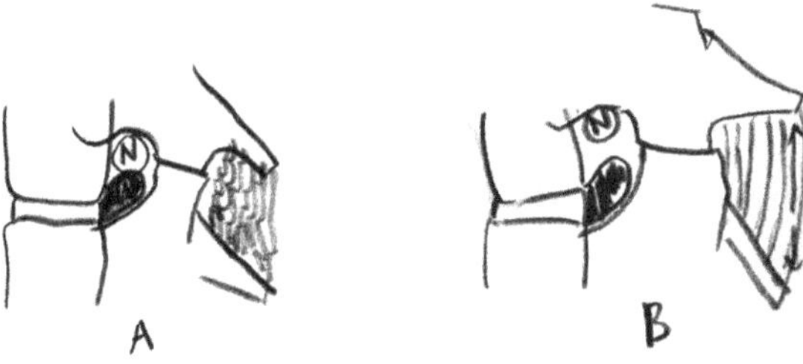

Figure 28-4. Kyphosis may be a temporary process occuring before the onset of disc degeneration. In the above figure a, on the left, a disc herniation (solid) is compressing the nerve (labelled N). As the disc height is unchanged by an acute disc herniation, voluntary flexion of the neck results in an increase in the size of the neural foramen, relieving pain and neurologic symptoms of nerve compression.

29 What is Cervical Spondylosis ?

Spondylosis is a general term used by radiologists and medical professionals describing a number of processes that occur during spinal degeneration. Using one common theory, the cervical disc begins any day with a maximum water saturated, which gives it a maximum volume and disc height. Subsequently, the pressure of load-bearing in an upright person results in the slow loss of water and height from the disc space. Like a rechargeable battery, over time, the disc does not fully reabsorb all of the water each day, and over time, loses height (degenerates).[109] Following the loss of height, the stabilizing ligaments, facet joint capsules, and disc annulus are no longer under tension, and they buckle. At this point, the disc space becomes less stable and is free to translate, or move anteriorly and posteriorly to a small extent. As a response to these additional forces, ligaments such as the interspinous and interlaminar ligaments will thicken as a result of the natural response to increased stress (Fig. 29-1). Following that, with enough erosing of the disc space and facet capsule , increased bone-on-bone forces result in a stress response that occurs in the bone. The end result of the stress response is the thickening of the bone (sclero-

---

109 *See chapter 22 regarding the process of cervical disc degeneration.*

sis), and then the projection of the bone to increase the surface area of contact.[110] When the bone adjacent to the disc develops projections, this is called an osteophyte, or bone spur. Also occurring when the disc collapses is bulging of the outward as the disc flattens. Disc herniations may also occur. Facet joints do not typically produce osteophytes, they enlarge, which is referred to as facet hypertrophy. The end result of these processes is a smaller neural foramen for the nerve (*N*, in figure) to exit the spine, which eventually can cause nerve compression.

---

110 *Osteophytes increase the surface area where forces are transmitting from one spinal level to the level below, and that decreases the pressure across the surface, and can eventually stabilize the spinal level over time—and in some cases, bone grows across the disc space, fusing the two levels (commonly referred to as autofusion).*

Spondylosis and Neural Foraminal Stenosis

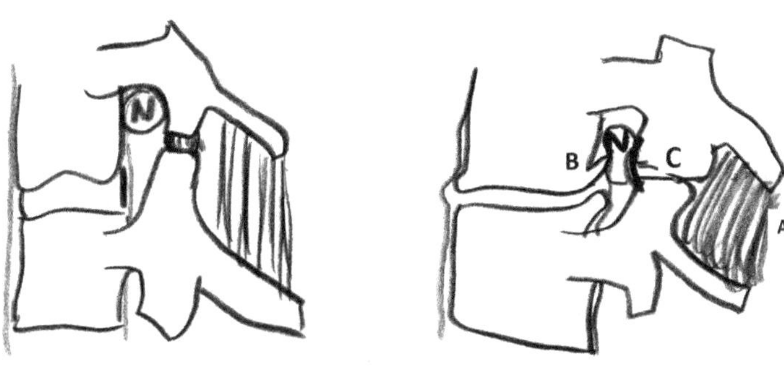

Figure 29-1. Cervical Spondylosis is a natural process of spinal degeneration of the hydrated cevical disc (Figure, image on left). Over time, the disc loses water and collapses, resulting in a loss of height not only for the disc (right image), but for the nerve (N) as well through a decrease in the ceiling of the neural foramen. Subsequently, additional motion occurs at this level as the ligaments are no longer under tension. This can cause ligamentous hypertrophy (A), where the ligaments thicken to handle the demands of the additional stress. Further contributing to the stenosis are the combination of osteophyte formation of the disc (B) and facet hypertrophy, which is enlargement of the two facet joints (labeled C). Also at point B, the disc can bulge into the spinal canal and also cause further narrowing at the neural foramen, where the nerve is seen exiting (labeled N). The overall result shown here cervical spondylosis resulting in cervical foraminal stenosis, which is the sum of all of those processes encroaching on the nerve root. Also, the central canal narrows as well and spinal cord compression can result (not shown).

30 How Is 'Arthritis' Described On The Spine Imaging Report?

The term arthritis is an almost universal term, but in the spine it is analgous to spondylosis.[111] This section contains a concise summary table of the different terms that are often encountered in a cervical imaging report. Remember that an imaging report is not a validation of the cause of symptoms, it is a description of the imaging report (ie. *CT or* MRI).

111 *For a detailed explanation of spondylosis, see chapter 28. For further detail regarding the various processes related to spondylotic conditions, see Chapter 22 regarding disc degeneration, 23-24 regarding disc herniations, and 25 regarding stenosis.*

Spinal Imaging Terminology

Facet arthropathy	Inflammation in the facet joints, where there are two per level in the lumbar spine. These joints facilitate motion.
Spurs (osteophytes)	A sign of chronic 'wear and tear'. The body develops these bone spurs to distribute forces evenly through a disc level and to stabilize abnormal motion.
Degenerative disc	Loss of water and collagen in the disc, resulting in decreased space between the vetebra.
Modic changes	Describes inflammation in the bone adjacent to the degenerated disc (the end-plate).
Ligamentous hypertrophy	Ligaments thickening, that occurs in response to abnormal motion at a 1 or many levels of the spine.
Stenosis	Narrowing of a space or channel, and in the spine this can cause compression of a nerve root.

31 What is Cervical Scoliosis?

Cervical scoliosis is usually mild, and most often just a curious finding on an imaging report. Because it is relatively rare compared to thoracic and lumbar scoliosis, it is not listed in the previous chapter. When the spine is viewed from the front, an imaginary line should expect the spine to be straight. Normally, the head should always be centered over the pelvis, as any deviation to the left or right asymmetrically loads the spine and extremities to maintain balance. Over time, for a myriad of reasons, degeneration can occur preferentially on one side of the disc, resulting in uneven loading of the spine, and accelerated disc degeneration in an asymmetric manner. This can result in curvature of the spine, and has been reported to occur to some degree in 68% of adults over 60 in the lumbar spine.[112] This process of degenerative scoliosis does not

---

112 *Schwab F, et al. Adult scoliosis: prevalence, SF-36, and nu-*

readily occur in the cervical spine as there is much less weight supported by the cervical spine, and the joints of the neck are less accomodating to developing this curvature.

Cervical Scoliosis Compensation Secondary to Thoracic and Lumbar Scoliosis

Thoracic and lumbar scoliosis is more frequent than cervical scoliosis, and when encountered on imaging, it is usually the result of the bodies attempt to balance use the cervical and upper thoracic spine to maintain the center of gravity over the pelvis (Fig. 31-1). Cervical scoliosis is exceedingly rare, and is encountered most often in genetic conditions, many of which are associated with genetic syndromes.[113]

Observations of Curvature Usually Do Not Meet the Requirements To cause Significant Stenosis

To classify a patient as having scoliosis, many academic and professional surgeon societies have designated a minimal curvature of ten degrees to meet the criteria, but this is traditionally set forth for the thoracic and lumbar spine. Your report usually defines scoliosis as any curvature (1 degree or greater). This measurent, called the Cobb Angle, is meant to be performed in a standard manner, but variations in measurement do occur, and are based on the experience of the facility taking the measurement.[114]

---

tritional parameters in an elderly volunteer population. Spine. 2005 30(9):1082-5.

113 *Singh H, Ghobrial G, Harrop J. Scoliotic Cervical Deformity. Spine Surgery: Techniques, Complication Avoidance, and Management (3rd &4th Edition). Editor: Edward C. Benzel.*

114 *For more information in depth on the Cobb Angle: https://radiopaedia.org/articles/cobb-angle?lang=us*

Cervical Scoliosis Is Usually Incidental and Compensatory[115]

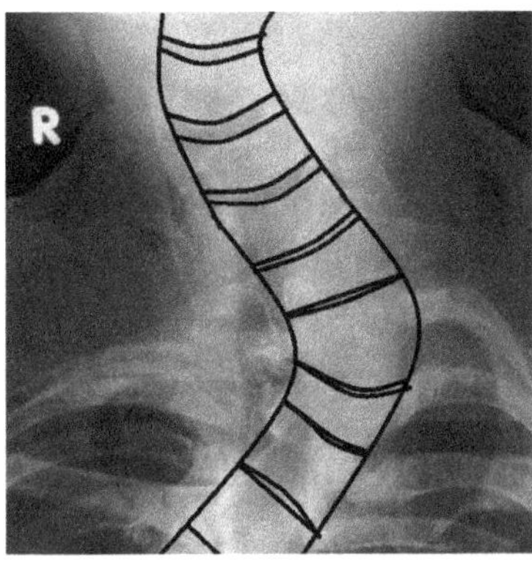

Figure 31-1. Cervical scoliosis when encountered in an adult, is usually very mild, resulting from cervical compensatory changes (Curvature of cervical changes outlined on radiograph) to balance the center of gravity which is affected by mild thoracic or lumbar scoliosis (curvature labeled B). Scoliosis is a three-dimensional curvature and an AP film alone can underestimate the magnitude of the curve. Conceptualize this by rotating a coat hanger and observing the curvature of the shadow from a flashlight.

Most Patients With Scoliosis Do Not Require Surgery

Most people with radiographic scoliosis do not end up requiring surgery. For complex and uncommon issues such as cervical scoliosis, which can be compensatory, genetic, and for a number of other uncommon reasons, an individualized approach will be taken. It is best to seek expert evaluation early as significant cervical scoliosis can cause thoracic and lumbar symptoms that may not improve, or in turn can be a secondary manifestation of other

115 *Incidental - Often seen on an imaging Study, and even with patients without symptoms. Often of limited to no significance, or a sign of mild thoracic scoliosis, and therefore a compensation (compensatory) to realign your center of gravity. When the term compensatory is used, it is not as in 'compensatory damages.'*

issues impacting your overall balance. This can lead to intractable pain and a poor quality of life.

How Does Scoliosis Worsen Quality of Life?

The body senses prolonged curvature as abnormal stress, which responds in the same way as the process of spondylosis. Once again, for the above reasons, curvature in the spine can develop, most commonly from a disc degnerating asymmetrically in the thoracic or lumbar spine, or in the case of the cervical spine as a compensation secondary to the development of thoracic or lumbar scoliosis. The process of progression of the scoliosis can cause unilateral narrowing of the neuroforamina (Fig. 31-2) on the inside of the curve, also called the concavity. Enlargement of the facet joints, thickening of the ligaments, or disc bulging can then occur as a result of scoliosis, causing stenosis and nerve compression.

Cervical Forminal Stenosis Resulting from Cervical Scoliosis

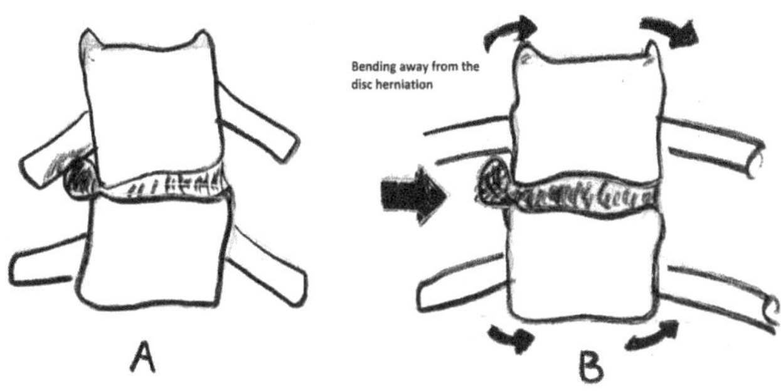

Figure 31-2. Cervical Scoliosis may contribute to stenosis. In the normal cervical spine, there is an even 'height' and the nerves exit between pedicles, and underneath the facet joints . Curvature results in increased space on the outside of the curve, and decreased space on the inside of the curve, further compounded when a disc herniation occurs (A). Bending away from the disc herniation can provide relief, as seen here (Figure B).

Surgery For Cervical Scoliosis Is Rare, and Involves Decompression And Fusion

Scoliosis is a progressive problem. Symptoms can manifest as increased fatigue, back pain, and then other symptoms from nerve compression. The surgical management of cervical scoliosis is complex. However, it may illustrate the purpose of spinal instrumentation in a fusion procedure.

As the spine begins to curve, new forces are directed laterally, which in addition to the force exerted by your body mass results in curve progression, followed by thickening of bone. Decompression of the nerves in this situation, just like with cervical subluxation, results in not only decompressing a nerve but in removing the stabilizing components. In the thoracic and lumbar spine, decompression of the exiting spinal nerves without the need for stabilization with screws and rods has been shown to be effective in many patients in which there was minimal slippage of one vertebral body beyond the adjacent level (lateral listhesis), and limited rotation of the vertebra.[116] However, in the cervical spine, patients with abnormal loss of cervical lordosis and scoliosis, posterior stabilizing fusion is recommended.[117]

Preventing worsening cervical scoliosis after decompression surgery requires spinal stabilization with screws, rods, or other stabilizing technologies as indicated by your surgeon. The process of fusion occurs over months as bone bridges the operative levels. Stabilizing the spine means eliminating motion at those levels. As previously mentioned, the management of scoliosis is individualized and complex, and is out of the scope of this guide.

---

116 *Kelleher MO et al. Success and failure of minimally invasive decompression for focal lumbar lspinal stenosis in patients with and without deformity. Spine 25(19): 2010.*

117 *Kim BS et al. Cervical laminectomy: with or without lateral mass instrumentation: A Comparison of OUtcomes. Clin Spine Surg. 32(6):226-232, 2019.*

SECTION IV

NON-SURGICAL TREATMENT

32 Which Medications Relieve Neck Pain?

Acute neck pain is a very common condition caused by **muscle strain**, a painful inflammatory process of the muscles, that is caused by overuse, stretching, and 'microtears' of the muscle. In other words, this is an overuse injury of the muscle. The varying levels of injury range from simple overuse and temporary discomfort lasting a few days to a week to permanent discomfort due to muscular tears. For people that enjoy lifting weights or bodybuilding, this might be a more common experience, especially earlier on when certain muscles (shoulder girdle) are activated more by certain motions not currently encountered in usual 'activities of daily living'(Fig. 32-1).

Neck Musculature Involved In Acute Muscle Strain

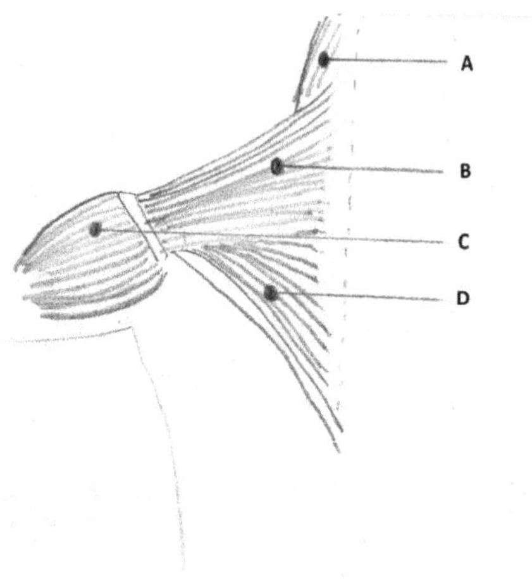

Figure 32-1. The common neck muscles involved in acute muscle strain are illustrated above in a depiction of the upper shoulder girdle and neck muscles from a posterior view of the left side: the sternocleidomastoid(A), The trapezius (B), rhomboids (major and minor groups are located deep to the trapezius, C), and the deltoids (D).

Commonly activated muscles include the deltoids, trapezius, rhomboids, erector spinae, and sternocleidomastoid. Muscular conditioning decreases the chances of muscular strain and shortens the recovery period. Novice weightlifters may recall the first time they targeted the shoulder girdle muscles. Bodybuilders and other athletes who target these muscle groups frequently are at risk of painful muscular strain. When muscle recovers from strain, the inflammatory process is anabolic, and results in a stronger, more conditioned muscle. The process of bodybuilding is to target muscles to failure, but without causing injury. For most people, neck pain is caused by prolonged neck positioning where certain muscles are consistently activated and over-exerted. It is easy to identify these conditions when the neck neck is persistently extended or flexed (Fig. 32-2).

Prolonged Extension and Flexion Loads The Neck Musculature, Contributing To Muscle Strain

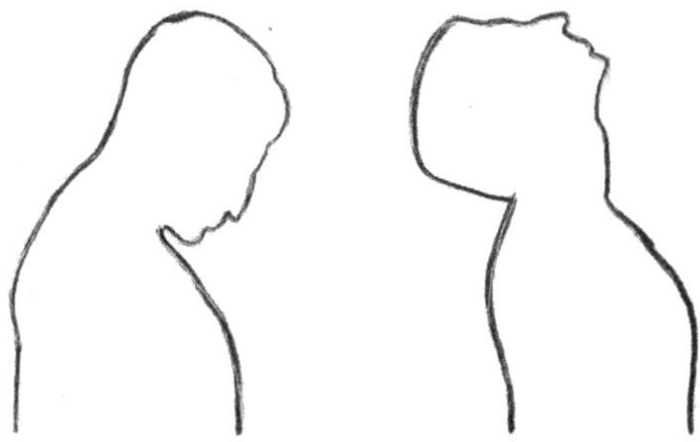

Figure 32-2. Neck extension and Flexion Contribute to Neck Pain. Prolonged Flexion (left image) of the neck places posterior neck muscles under maximum stretch and tension, while similarly neck extension (right image) places anterior neck muscles under maximum stretch and prolonged contraction of the posterior neck musculature occurs. Both states of porlonged flexion and extension cause abnormal loading of the cervicothoracic junction.

Ergonomics and Neck Pain

Poor posture can cause back and neck pain. One area may stand out above else, and that is how we position our body at work. This is referred to as **ergonomics**. People in general prefer to have the object that we are looking at in the center of our field of view, while looking horizontally (Fig. 32-3). Also, neutral neck positioning is vital to avoid placing the neck into constant flexion or extension, as in the above figure.

Improper workplace ergonomics is a very common example where neck pain, among other health issues if you are not attentive to how your monitor is set up. Often the most common example is that the computer monitor is lower than your head, placing the center of the screen below your natural field of view, which is horizontal, which requires your neck to be neutral (Fig. 32-4).

Workplace Ergonomics Can Prevent Acute and Chronic Neck Pain

To keep the object of interest centered, flexing our neck and to a lesser degree increasing thoracolumbar kyphosis (hunching over') lowers the head and centers the area of interest (the most common area of interest at the desk is the computer monitor (Fig. 32-3).

Proper Workplace Ergonomics

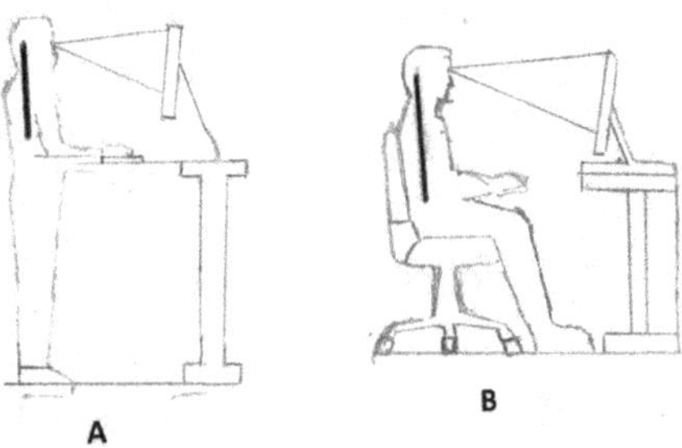

Figure 32-3. Appropriate Ergonomics can prevent neck pain. In these figures, appropriate positioning of the monitor has been achieved both at a standing desk (A), or with office chair, through adjustment of the height of the monitor (B). This way, the position of the head is centered over the pel-

vis while maintaining a neutral cervicothoracic spine, as delineated by the straight lines above.

Improper Workplace Ergonomic: One Example

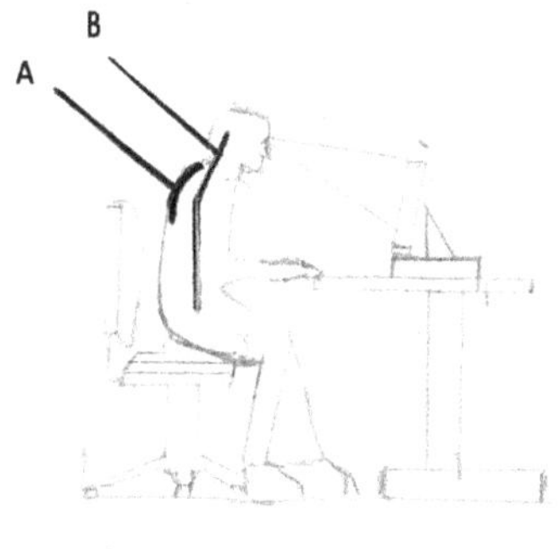

Figure 32-4. Improper attention to ergonomics is all too common. Seen above, this diligent worker is attempting to maintain his appropriate horizontal gaze, which is still slightly below horizontal. The head is slightly flexed, the thoracic kyphosis is increased (A), and the cervicothoracic alignment is no longer neutral (B). Prolonged positioning like this can lead to neck and low back pain.

In the author's opinion, multiple changes occur all over the body to decrease the energy demand and workload on one joint/region to allow for a less strenuous compensation. It would be unlikely that the eyes are redirected to an area out of our center field because it is very exhausting on the eyes. Frankly, prolonged gaze to the periphery causes eye strain, and is painful. As an exercise, you can try and see how long you can look as far to the left, right, up or down while keeping your head and body stationary. Note that it's tough to do for more than a few seconds and is not comfortable.

Anti-inflammatory Medications Are Ideal For Muscle Strain, an Inflammatory Process

At the cellular level, muscle strain refers to cellular trauma or muscle injury ('microtears') which causes inflammation of the muscle. Inflammatory signalling triggers local swelling, resulting in creased white blood cells at the site of injury, and the white blood cells release more signalling molecules that can cause redness and pain. While the process of inflammation is a natural process of healing, it is the swelling, redness, and pain that affects our perception of well-being and ultimately our daily functioning. Anti-inflammatory medications are highly affective as a pain reliever by blocking inflammatory pathways.

Over the counter (OTC) anti-inflammatory medications are a class of medication known as a non-steroidal anti-inflammatory drug (NSAID), and are ideal in that they are effective, not habit forming, and when taken for short time periods, the OTC forms of NSAIDS have a limited side-effect profile. The most common NSAID is ibuprofen, which targets inflammation. Acetaminophen, is not classified as an NSAID and does not target the anti-inflammatory pathways as ibuprofen. However, these medications are the most recommended for acute neck pain. Oral corticosteroids are occasionally prescribed for short durations for severe neck pain that does not improve with NSAIDs. Some patients state that they have experienced near complete relief of neck pain with a short course of steroids, serving as furthur indirect evidence of the manner at which basic inflammatory pathways mediate painful muscular strain. Oral corticosteroids negatively impact organ systems, and is a dangerous tool, that only grows more dangerous with each successive dose. **Prolonged use of any medication can will lead to adverse effects, even with the most 'innocuous' medications such as NSAIDs.** Abuse of acetaminophen and ibuprofen beyond recommended dosages and durations carry risks of serious medical complications, including but not limited injury to the liver and kidneys, respectively.

Anti-inflammatory medications are recommended early on within 1 month of onset, and the chronic use of NSAIDs carry an increased risks of side-effects. In one prospective study, of the 249 patients followed, the average duration of neck pain was 16 days, with most patients stating that pain lasted under 6 weeks.[118] Most of these patients were therefore able to manage their neck pain with OTC medications.

Ibuprofen Is Preferable To Acetaminophen For Neck Pain

Overall, low-quality evidence limits the recommendation of acetaminophen or ibuprofen in favor of one or the other.[119] Acetaminophen is generally recognized as having much less anti-inflammatory activity than ibuprofen as acetaminophen is a weak inhibitor of key inflammatory enzyme mediators, cyclooxygenase 1 and 2. And while this has been shown in a lab setting, there is no clear superior medication because of the lack of high quality research studies comparing the two.

A meta-analysis is a scientific attempt to summarize the results of many studies, large and small, in an attempt to draw greater conclusions than possible with a single study. One study, by Enthoven[120] found NSAIDs to be more effective than no treatment at all, for low back pain. More data exists for the treatment of osteoarthritis, which found five of seven randomized controlled trials

---

118 *Vos C et al. Management of Acute Neck Paick In General Practice: A prospective Study. British Journal Of General Practice, Jan. 2007.*

119 *Botting RM. Mechanism of Action of Acetaminophen: Is There a Cyclooxygenase 3? Clinical Infectious Disease. 31(suppl 5):S202-210; 2000.*

120 *Enthoven WT et al. Non-steroidal anti-inflammatory drugsd for chronic low back pain. Cochrane Database Syst Rev. 2(2): 2016.*

to show a significant advantage of ibuprofen over acetaminophen in terms of pain reduction and limiting side effects.[121] A cautionary approach is recommended when interpreting studies that attempt to summate other research. Many studies are dissimilar enough in terms of study design, research quality, patient population characteristics, and innumerable other details that a reasonable summation of the research is not possible. Moreover, the two studies were used as examples to illustrate the effectiveness of the medications, but must be taken with a grain of salt as they do not specifically study the use of ibuprofen for short durations of acute neck pain.

Key Points

- Although variations in clinical practice occur due to limited high quality research on acute neck pain, prescription analgesics (opiates) are not recommended for acute neck pain.

- Explore all of your options with your physician or healthcare provider, who likely has tremendous experience in neck pain care, as it is among the most common reasons for patients to seek attention at his or her primary care office.

- Understand the risks of all medications that you take. The major NSAID side-effects involve but are not limited to the GI symptoms (from absorption of the medication), hypertension, and elimination of the medication (kidney or liver).

- Once again, avoid opiate use.

---

121 *Towheed et al. Acetaminophen For Osteoarthritis. Cochrane Database Syst Rev. 2006.*

Differences Between Acetaminophen and Ibuprofen

- Acetaminophen is primarily a pain-reliever, and not technically an NSAID, and has very little anti-inflammatory properties
- Ibuprofen is an anti-inflammatory medication (NSAID), whereas acetaminophen is not.
- Of the OTC medications, NSAIDs will be most helpful in relieving symptoms driven by inflammation.

Muscle Relaxants For Neck Pain

Muscle relaxers are another option that may help with pain control secondary to painful muscle spasms. Some medical evidence shows that skeletal muscle relaxants improve short term pain when compared to placebo (compared to no treatment). Also, there is not much support for one muscle relaxant over another. Most muscle relaxants do not work primarily on the muscle cells themselves, but rather, they target the central nervous system, mostly in the brain, causing additional affects, such as intoxicating effects. They should not be used in conjunction with opiates, or other medications that target the CNS except under the close direction of an experienced physician as the perceived adverse effects are much greater.

33 What Should I Try During the First Months of Symptoms?

There are numerous treatment options in the first month of acute neck pain. Since most acute neck pain improves spontaneously after 2-4 weeks, it is common practice to begin with the least invasive options and those with the lowest risk profile first. As a result, the most common recommendations early on for acute neck pain include heat, ice, NSAIDs, and physical therapy.

There are numerous other options as well, which are thought to be helpful for any form of back or neck pain. It is difficult to compare and contrast treatments and provide a scientific study comparing treatments because the diagnostic process for the underlying causes of acute neck pain is less precise. Once again, MRI studies of the neck may identify disc deneration, herniation, perhaps suggest inflammation in the neck muscles, and highlight other spondylotic processes, but this is far from what physicians refer to as a 'definitive diagnosis'. Therefore, recognize that acute neck pain is incredibly common, most often not due to a concerning process warranting immediate MRI workup, and in many studies resolves in the majority of patients treated between 3 and 12 months.[122] **Choosing the most effective neck pain treatment may be a trial-and-error process.** Again, it is often hard to distinguish the normal improvement in neck pain from an effect of a given treatment. This is because most acute neck pain improves without seeking treatment.

The options listed below are excellent because they are shown to be helpful in alleviating low back pain. Since low back pain can often spontaneously improve, it is sometimes hard to know if low back pain improvement occurred due to the treatment, or if this was just going to happen anyway. As a result, if there are no red flag symptoms, it is adviseable to consider the therapies below, or generally any therapy that has a low risk profile, and is a non-invasive procedure.

---

122 *Cecchi F, Predictors of short- and long-term outcome in patients with chronic non-specific neck pain undergoing an exercise-based rehabilitation program: a prospective cohort study with 1-year follow-up. Intern Emerg Med. 6(5):413-21, 2011.*

Common First Line Treatments For Neck Pain[123]

Common First Line Treatments For Neck Pain
Physical Therapy
Stretching and Light exercise
Spinal Manipulation Therapy (Chiropractic manipulation)
Ice
Heat
OTC Anti-inflammatory Medications
Chiropracter
Accupuncture
Massage
Dry Needling
Meditation
Yoga and Tai Chi
Meditation and Stress Reduction
Aquatherapy
Application of Heat or Ice

123 *Observe caution with any therapies that involve traction on the neck. Spinal manipulation of the neck, and any therapy applying force to the neck carries the potential risk damage to the arteries of the neck, which can cause life threatening stroke. For further details on this very rare complication, see Biller J et al. Cervical arterial dissections and association with cervical manipulative therapy: a statement for healthcare professionals from the American Heart Association/American Stroke Association. Stroke. 45(10):3155-2174, 2014.*

34 When Is it Safe To Return to Work?

This is a very common question asked by patients in a spine clinic. **The answer to this question all depends on numerous factors such as the requirements of the job and your specific clinical history.** Moreover, there are many obstacles to obtaining a straight answer to this question. Some patients ask this question about returning to work (RTW), while some patients ask this question because their employer requires some form of clearance. In that regard, most spine experts are not experts at the intricacies of work safety, and are not aware of the unique requirements of the countless occupations and their respective requirements and hazards.

Hypothetical Example: The F-15 Pilot At The National Guard— Return To Work

To use a purely hypothetical example, a patient with neck pain has degenerative disc disease, which began as a sharp pain in the morning, shortly after waking up 4 weeks ago. Since then, the pain has been improving— However, for the purposes of advancing this hypothetical example, the patient requires that the physician authorize a clearance to 'return to work'. This healthy-young man is 35 and denies any other concerning medical symptoms or history. He is an F-15 pilot who flies several hours a day, 3-5 days per week, with the local national guard. After discussing the extent of neck pain, no imaging is required.

Although there is no medical reason identified to limit this patient's return to work, most would agree that this is an exotic occupation, which has unique considerations, most of which are unknown to most people, outside of a military base, and a military facility, who are aware that an F-15 may be able to fly upwards of 1875 miles per hour.

In most other people, all that can be said from above example is that degenerative disc disease (DDD) is normally found in most imaging, and it is difficult to link neck pain to DDD and by itself does not serve as an exclusion to any activity. Moreover, very little insight can be gained from the medical literature and a physician's personal experience with fighter pilots with neck pain (outside of a military hospital or clinic).[124]

---

124 *Incidentally, for those interested about pilots. Cervical degenerative disc disease was not noted to be more prevalent in the aircraft pilot population. This review of the published medical literature did find a small correlation between acute neck pain and high-performance aircraft pilots, but overall this serves as a weak correlation. Shiri R. et al. Cervical and lumbar pain and radiological degeneration among fighter pilots: a system-*

As a general rule, for most neck pain problems due to disc degeneration of the cervical spine without neurologic deficits, discussions about return to work for most cases are usually limited. **The finding on MRI of degenerative disc disease, in isolation of any other clinical findings, a finding that exists in most people in their forties and fifties, would not be expected to disqualify them from working.** Guidance pertaining to further requirements usually reside with one's employer and their specific requirements for returning to work.

Neck Pain with Neurologic Symptoms

On the other hand, spinal cord injury or nerve compression causing weakness or numbness, and other specific findings, is a specific consideration that would require further assessment.
The decision to return to work most likely will require an expert in spinal disorders (see your healthcare provider) and someone who can perform a functional capacity evaluation. Inquire with your physician to determine if that is part of their training, which is to provide a standardized evaluation of one's disability, often expressed as a percentile. Often, employers want to know what a person's percent disability is related to a medical issue, and this if often in reference to an assessment of functional capacity. Again, this is a service that not all healthcare providers provide, is time consuming, utilizes staff members in an office to complete lengthy documentation, and as a result this is confined to larger practice settings. Therefore, you will often have to inquire further regarding this subject.

---

atic review and meta-analysis. Occup Environ Med. 72(2):145-50, 2014.

35 What Medications Should I Avoid Early On?

There is no specific rule about which medications should be avoided, just general guidelines. However, be extremely cautious of the addictive potential of prescription pain relievers, and their negative effects. This cannot be overstated. Drug overdoses are now the leading cause of death in the U.S. for people under age 55.[125]

125 *'Heroin addiction explained: How opioids Hijack the Brain, NY Times Dec 18, 2018*

How Can My Risk For Opiate Addiction be Assessed?

One helpful tool used by physicians to assess for addiction potential in the setting of chronic pain is the opiate risk tool (ORT). A list of the opiates being prescribed and their relative strengths, effectiveness, and potency will be listed in the following section.

Opioid Risk Tool

Opioid Risk Tool		
	Female	**Male**
Family history		
Alcohol abuse	1	3
Prescription drug abuse	2	3
Illicit drug use	4	4
Personal History		
Alcohol abuse	3	3

Prescription drug abuse	4	4
Illicit drug use	5	5
Age 16-45?	1	1
History of preadolescent sexual abuse?	3	0
Psychiatric History?	2	2
Depression	1	1

Use the ORT above and use the table below to calculate the total score:

Score	Risk
<4	Low
4-7	Moderate risk
>7	High

36 Opiates Are The Last Resort

Opiates are really not effective for chronic pain. Also, opiate use is generally not a first-line therapy for short term pain. Regardless of how severe acute pain might be, opiates are generally not recommended for acute pain. All other medications and therapies should be attempted before taking opiates. From the point of one's first exposure to opiates (eg. hydrocodone, oxycodone) the body quickly builds tolerance to the medication, and the medication quickly loses effectiveness in treating pain. As the body becomes more tolerant, one can become addicted, and in some patients, they become more sensative to pain.

Why does the body adjust in such a way to opiate exposure? It is not entirely clear, but one theory is that the body modifies pain according to its environment, as a way to protect the body from harm's way. Avoiding dangerous environmental exposure (eg. extreme hot or cold), after all, is a basic function of survival and procreation. If opiates decrease or block pain signals to your brain altogether on a daily basis, some researchers theorize that the brain can automatically increases your sensitivity to pain signals (like turning the 'gain' up on a stereo). This is to make sure one is aware of the painful stimuli that one should be avoiding. Regardless of how they exactly work, opiates are the last resort and should be avoided if at all possible.

Key Points

- This can't be overstated, opiates are a last resort medication.

- Avoid opiate prescriptions at all costs in the first three months for acute back and neck pain, if possible. Every medical society with guidelines for opiate use is in agreement with this statement. There are exceptions, and these can be discussed with a physician (eg. cancer).

- Before considering opiates, see if one has improvement with either: NSAIDs, muscle relaxers, glucocorticoids (steroids), benzodiazepines, nerve membrane stabilizers and just about any non-opiate class of medication before considering opiates.

Brief List of Common Opiate Medications

Medication (drug name)	Common Trade Name (tm)	Strength	Acetaminophen Formulations Available
Codeine	Tylenol-Codeine (No. 3/No. 4)	+	Yes
Hydrocodone	Vicodin/Norco (contains acetaminophen)	++	Yes
Oxycodone	Oxycontin, Roxicodone	+++	Yes
Hydromorphone	Dilaudid	++++	No
Fentanyl	Duragesic	++++	No
Buprenorphine/naloxone	Suboxone	+++	No
Methadone	Dolophine, Methadose	++++	No

Common Opiate prescription drugs with trade name and potency.

Opiates - Key Points

Below you will find some brief comments about the preceding list of opiates that may be of some use to You.

- Treat them all as equals. While they vary in potency, time of onset, duration of effect, route, and risk of adverse effects, a prescription for codeine, hydrocodone, and oxycodone can potentially lead to an escalating addiction problem. There is no such thing as a short trial of opiates- which is among the most common circumstances by which chronically addicted patients first become introduced to opiates.

- Be aware of the presence of acetaminophen in select opiates. There is enough acetaminophen in these medications that chronic, intermittent daily use can lead to irreversible liver injury. The upper limit of daily acetamnophen use has decreased over time. It is understood that 4,000 mg as an upper limit may still be toxic to some people. There is enough that is unknown about acetaminophen, and how body weight plays a role in safe liver doses, that it is recommended to stay below 3,000 mg per day if at all possible.[126]

- Avoid opiate usage with other medications that act on the central nervous system (CNS). Opiates taken with CNS-acting medications can often lead to far greater CNS suppression than expected (a synergistic effect). One-third of opiate overdoses occurred with the simultaneous use of benzodizepines. Benzodiazepines are a sedative used for anxiety, and often as a muscle relaxant. They work by increasing inhibitory

---

126 *https://www.health.harvard.edu/pain/acetaminophen-safety-be-cautious-but-not-afraid*

neurotransmitters in the brain, and not directly on the muscle. Most muscle relaxants work by targeting the brain to produce the effect of mucle relaxation.

- Codeine: This is among the weakest of the opiates, and can be found in tablets and cough suppressants.

- Short acting medications: Immediate release medications carry a relatively greater risk for adverse effects such as oversedation and respiratory suppression.

- Extended-release medications: Help to increase the duration of effect for opiates, which typically provide pain relief for very short durations. They achieve this extended effect by a manufactured process that delays absorption. In summary, follow the instructions from the pharamist precisely. These drugs usually say, "Do Not Chew", which allows them to provide extended duration of pain relief by slowly absorbing the medication into your blood.

- Fentanyl is highly potent and involved in nearly half of opiate-related deaths. It is appropriate for use predominantly in a hospital setting where it is given intravenously or ocasionally as a patch that is absorbed across your skin.

- Opioid dependence is a situation where a body will require a certain dose of an opioid to prevent withdrawl symptoms.

- Opioid addiction, is generally known as substance use disorder, which includes the psychiatric components of dependence.

- Methadone is used to treat opioid addiction. It has a delayed onset of action and for this reason does not produce the same degree of euphoria as heroin, morphine, and fentanyl. This drug is administered through drug abuse treatment centers ('methadone clinics').

- Buprenorphine/Naloxone (Suboxone) is similar in the intended effect as methadone, but far less potent of a medication. It is used for chronic pain, and unlike methadone, it can be prescribed by physicians for use outside of drug abuse treatment centers. If Suboxone were to be injected, naloxone would bind to the opioid receptors to prevent a delayed and lessened euphoria.

37 **What Are the Dangers of Opiates?**

Opiates killed over 70,000 Americans in 2017. Opioid overdose is the leading cause of death under the age of 55. This is due to either prescription or illicit drug use and fentanyl/fentanyl analogues, a very potent and fast acting opiate accounts for about 40% of these deaths. Death most often results from respiratory failure from overdose. Normal exposure to opiates decreases your rate of breathing. As your tolerance level increases, this respiratory suppression increases to levels that your body cannot adapt to. These medications are even more dangerous when used in combination with other prescription medications, or with alcohol use as the effects are far greater.

Key Points

The following is a very brief summary highlighting only some of the most dangerous adverse effects of opiates, and a discussion of the risks of constipation, nausea, and urinary retention with opiates will more than likely occur in your PCP office:

Addiction

Opioids are highly addicting, but limited research available shows that the potential for abuse varies highly from one person to the next.[127] Close to 10% of those taking opioids develop temporary addictive behaviors or permanent addiction. Rather than attempting to understand one's potential for addiction, it would be safer to assume that this risk should not be downplayed. To assess one's own risk, risk assessment tools for opiate abuse are used by clinicians to be aware of higher risk groups of patients (Chapter 34).

Withdrawal

This can still be fatal, but far less severe relative to opiate overdose. Opiate withdrawal can Long term use increases the risk of withdrawal symptoms if opiate reduction isn't planned carefully. Withdrawal can be experienced in as early as 4 to 6 hours, and occurs in most after 10 hours.[128]

---

127 *Dunn KE et al. Individual differences in human opioid abuse potential as observed in a human laboratory study. Drug Alcohol Depend. Dec 1;205:107688, 2019*

128 *Dunn K et al. Differences in patient-reported and observer -rated*

Tolerance

The body can become increasingly tolerant with prolonged use. The opiates quickly lose their efficacy and in all patients using opiates it is not long before greater doses are required to achieve the same effect. There is no known maximum opiate dose when the doses are slowly increased over time, as the body can become tolerant to the CNS side-effects with time.

Respiratory Suppression

One of the most concerning effects is that decreased breathing occurs with higher doses, which can be fatal. It is estimated that 90 Americans die each day from an opioid overdose, and this is usually from respiratory arrest. Medications that are highly potent opiates such as fentanyl are a major cause of death due to the relative ease at which very high dosages can be accidentally administered. Other inhibtory medications that target the brain (central nervous system) can increase the effects of opiates. Benzodiazepines and alcohol can amplify the effects of opiate use and can cause life-threatening respiratory suppression.

Increased Sensitivity to Pain

This is the opposite of what you want opiates to do, and it happens, increasing your demand for more opiates. This is a component of what is seen with an increased tolerance, but what is

opioid withdrawal symptom etiology, time course, and relationship to clinical outcome. Drug Alcohol Depend. Aug,2020.

really happening is the efficacy is steadily decreasing due to tolerance and an increased sensitivity to pain.

In other words, long term use of opiates at high doses may increase the likelihood of developing a hypersensitivity syndrome. More recent research suggests that the activation of glial cells(cells of your nervous tissue) increases interleukin-1 beta expression (inflammatory marker) which has been shown to increase chronic pain. The brain does increase the intensity of pain signals after prolonged opioid use partly out of an adaptation to be able to sense environmental threats.

38 What are Some of the Things I Can Do to Decrease My Neck Pain Long Term?

There are a seemingly endless number of options for the treatment of neck pain. There are no quick fixes, regardless of how much one desires them. For most people, neck pain will come and go, regardless of any treatment and it is a very common problem. If the problem appears to be worsening, there are some other things to consider about how you can influence your quality of life.

Additionally, for people with neck AND arm pain, this problem will also go away after a few months without any invasive treatments. Some authors argue that strict routine and poor ergonomics are features of many chronic neck pain cases.

Below, some common therapies are listed that are considered beneficial for short term and long term neck pain reduction. Advanced imaging, such as magnetic resonance imaging of the lumbar spine(MRI) is not recommended for most people with neck pain, without meeting strict criteria. This is to help limit patients obtain unnecessary imaging studies, and to limit growing healthcare costs in North America.

Two Pitfalls With Early MRI and Neck Pain:[129]

- An MRI cannot link a specific 'finding' (a 'finding' is anything that the radiologist describes) with the cause of neck pain for most cases of a spinal degenerative process. Since neck pain is vague, and not specific to the disc levels, the facet joints, or muscles and ligaments.

- An MRI does not quantify spondylosis, or in another words, determine if the arthritic processes of the spine are age-appropriate or 'excessive'.

---

129 *This section is adapted From The Low Back Pain Handbook, with permission, Weatherly Press, 2019.*

General Options for the Treatment of Chronic or Recurrent Neck Pain

Weight loss
Core strengthening and physical therapy
Meditation
Stretching
Yoga
Massage
Aquatherapy
Tai Chi
TENS
Pharmacotherapy
Interventional Pain Management Techniques

39 How Does Weight Gain Cause Neck Pain?

Weight gain affects every system of the body— And before diving straight into the link between weight gain and neck pain, the question of abnormal weight and how weight is measured by healthcare professionals needs to be explained. One measurement system is the body-mass index (BMI), which allows height to be accounted for when assessing for for obesity (Fig. 39-1). The center for disease control (CDC) has an online measurement tool and other evidence-based learning tools as well for anyone interested in quickly assessing their BMI. Other tools that can be found on the CDC-site are guides for weight loss and maintenance. Information from the

CDC will not differ from the advice of most healthcare providers, and this site can spare one the hassle of navigating through additional private advertisements and other 'noise' associated with online calculators, which exist mainly to draw in business.[130] Using BMI, organized into groups, for example, 18.5-24.9, 25.0-29.9, and 30 and over correlating to normal, overweight, and obese, respectively, allow for researchers to more easily compare data across multiple research studies, and to provide concrete goals and cutoffs.

The BMI Index

	Normal						Overweight					Obese										Extreme Obesity						
BMI	19	20	21	22	23	24	25	26	27	28	29	30	31	32	33	34	35	36	37	38	39	40	41	42	43	44	45	46
Height (inches)	Body Weight (pounds)																											
58	91	96	100	105	110	115	119	124	129	134	138	143	148	153	158	162	167	172	177	181	186	191	196	201	205	210	215	220
59	94	99	104	109	114	119	124	128	133	138	143	148	153	158	163	168	173	178	183	188	193	198	203	208	212	217	222	227
60	97	102	107	112	118	123	128	133	138	143	148	153	158	163	168	174	179	184	189	194	199	204	209	215	220	225	230	235
61	100	106	111	116	122	127	132	137	143	148	153	158	164	169	174	180	185	190	195	201	206	211	217	222	227	232	238	243
62	104	109	115	120	126	131	136	142	147	153	158	164	169	175	180	186	191	196	202	207	213	218	224	229	235	240	246	251
63	107	113	118	124	130	135	141	146	152	158	163	169	175	180	186	191	197	203	208	214	220	225	231	237	242	248	254	259
64	110	116	122	128	134	140	145	151	157	163	169	174	180	186	192	197	204	209	215	221	227	232	238	244	250	256	262	267
65	114	120	126	132	138	144	150	156	162	168	174	180	186	192	198	204	210	216	222	228	234	240	246	252	258	264	270	276
66	118	124	130	136	142	148	155	161	167	173	179	186	192	198	204	210	216	223	229	235	241	247	253	260	266	272	278	284
67	121	127	134	140	146	153	159	166	172	178	185	191	198	204	211	217	223	230	236	242	249	255	261	268	274	280	287	293
68	125	131	138	144	151	158	164	171	177	184	190	197	203	210	216	223	230	236	243	249	256	262	269	276	282	289	295	302
69	128	135	142	149	155	162	169	176	182	189	196	203	209	216	223	230	236	243	250	257	263	270	277	284	291	297	304	311
70	132	139	146	153	160	167	174	181	188	195	202	209	216	222	229	236	243	250	257	264	271	278	285	292	299	306	313	320
71	136	143	150	157	165	172	179	186	193	200	208	215	222	229	236	243	250	257	265	272	279	286	293	301	308	315	322	329
72	140	147	154	162	169	177	184	191	199	206	213	221	228	235	242	250	258	265	272	279	287	294	302	309	316	324	331	338

Figure 39-1:The BMI Index Chart.(https://www.nhlbi.nih.gov/health/educational/lose_wt/BMI/bmi_tbl.htm)

130 *https://www.cdc.gov/healthyweight/assessing/bmi/adult_bmi/english_bmi_calculator/bmi_calculator.html*

While it is contended that these divisions are based on research, losing a single pound of weight to make one's BMI go from 'overweight' to 'normal' via a drop in BMI of 0.1 does not convince the author that the health risks have been nullified by so little of a change. Also, BMI is not appropriateas a marker for all, as those with high muscle mass and low body fat, such as bodybuilder-turned-actor Arnold Schwarzenegger (in his prime years), weighingover 200 lbs at a height of 6 foot 2 with very low bodyfat would still be classified as overweight. To counter this argument, most people have this problem. Some physicians measure waist size as some research correlates abdominal girth and waist circumference to the develpment of health problems such as diabetes and heart disease. Overall, it is likely that the risks of excessive weight are linear, and the appropriate mindset should focus more on limiting excess weight.

Another helpful government website is run by The National Heart, Lung, and Blood Institute (NHLBI), a division of the National Institute of Health (NIH), which is a research oriented site. For more detailed and specific information, the NHLBI site provides research and a range of other patient-oriented educational tools and links.[131]

As the main load-bearing support that allows us to stand upright, excess weight puts tremendous strain on the lumbar spine. Each spinal segment carries more weight, than the segment sitting above it. This explains why on average, the spinal segments become larger and larger as you progress from the first cervical segment to the fifth lumbar segment. As additional weight is gained, greater forces cause direct wear to the joints, which includes the disc, the facet joints, and a parallel process occurs where there is increased strain on the paraspinal muscles. Without the use of

---

131 *https://www.nhlbi.nih.gov/health-topics/overweight-and-obesity*

paraspinal muscles there would be no counter-balance to every bodily structure in front of the spine, such as the abdominal organs and fat. Studies have shown that significant weight loss helps lower low back and leg pain. In one study, patients with morbid obesity (BMI > 40) and low back pain underwent bariatric surgery, resulting in decreased leg pain. Patients were 270 pounds before, and 176 lbs after surgery.[132] It was observed in this study that patients had less low back and leg symptoms decreased, and the disc was measured as taller on follow-up imaging! This 2 millimeter increase is substantial (25% increase) and occasionally often enough to take the pressure fully off of a nerve, which was what was observed in the study. Small changes in weight have not been well studied, and the biggest changes have been shown in patients with a BMI over 35.[133]

How Does Neck Pain Result From Obesity?

The ideal posture is one where the head is centered over the feet, which uses the least amount of energy, keeping the body balanced, recruiting the least amount of muscle to keep the the spine balanced (Fig. 39-2). The spine, along with the pelvis, hips, knees, and ankles can flex or extend to help maintain the body's balance when standing upright. The regional segments of the spine: Lum-

---

132 *Bariatric surgery is surgery intended to subvert normal gastrointesional functioning in order to result in weight loss. This is accomplished through a less efficient absorption of calories, or early satiety. Both result in less calories taken in from a meal.*

133 *The Body-mass index (BMI) is a ratio of your weight to height. This is calculated most commonly with the formula for the metric system: Weight (kg) / (Height in meters)^2. Normal is considered between 18.5 to 24.9, Overweight is considered 25-29.9, and obesity is regarded as 30 and over. A formula for using pounds and inches: Weight (lbs) * 703 / (Height in inches)^2.*

bar, thoracic, and cervical can adjust by bending forward (flexion) or backward (extension). The overall purpose of this is to prevent the center of gravity from deviating away from the pelvis. Most often, the center of gravity shifts anteriorly due to the loss of lordosis of the lumbar spine, resulting in a center of gravity in front of the body. This is often seen with a combination of obesity, advanced lumbar degeneration, and a loss of lumbar lordosis. Decreased lordosis can lead to additional mechanisms of compensation by persistent extension of the neck, leading to chronic muscle strain, accelerated facet arthropathy and degeneration of the cervical spine. In addition, both low back and neck pain can occur on and off throughout these processes, and the absence does not indicate that these chronic spinal changes are not occuring. Low back and neck pain commonly occur together. [134] The relationship of simultaneous cervical and lumbar stenosis is very commonly observed, and thought to be related to the biomechanics of abnormal global spinal alignment. Also, increased abdominal weight can can result in the spine favoring a flexion of the lumbar spine (loss of lordosis) which results in increased stenosis in the lumbar spine, triggering the same global alignment problem above. There are numerous other relationships between neck pain and obesity but these illustrate the relationship.

---

134 *Baker JF. Evaluation and Treatment of Tandem Spinal Stenosis. J Am Acad Orthop Surg. 28(6):229-239, 2020.*

Neck Pain: A Result of Painful Compensation Measures Due to Abnormal Spinal Alignment Caused by Obesity

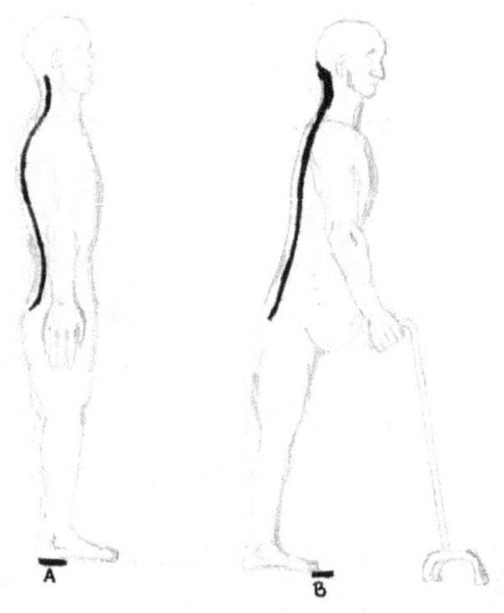

Figure 39-2. The Relationship Between Obesity and Neck Pain. Obesity can cause neck pain through a number of mechanisms. One way that obesity affects neck pain is through adversely shifting your center of gravity from the normal position over the pelvis(left image: center of gravity, A) to a strenuous position with a center of gravity in front of the feet (right image, spinal, pelvic, and lower extremity compensation to move the center of gravity closer to normal, B). Ultimately, the obesity results in straightening that cannot be easily compensated for, and many patients prefer a cane to assist with imbalance caused by an anterior center of gravity. As a result, postural changes in the thoracic and cervical spine occur which attempt to straighten the spine, moving the head closure to a position above the pelvis. These postural changes partially occur through increased strain on the paraspinal muscles. These abnormal changes in biomechanical forces can result in advanced degeneration of the cervical and thoracic spine. Obesity greatly accelerates degeneration of the lumbosacral spine, especially the discs, which are shock absorbers. As these discs lose height, the lumbar

spine loses lordosis. Also, a combination of changes results in stenosis. Symptomatic stenosis may result in the bodies tendency to lean forward, which has the effect of decreasing stenosis and relieving pressure on nerve roots. Both of these processes result in the lumbar spine losing lordosis and moving the whole body in a forward leaning posture, shifting the center of gravity forward. This is the start of one process where obesity leads to neck pain.

40 How Does Physical Therapy, Core Strengthening, and Exercise Conditioning Activities Help Non-Specific Neck Pain?

Many patients are surprised that physical therapy is a treatment for neck pain. In fact, neck pain is a very common recommendation, accounting for 25% of outpatient physical therapy (PT) referrals in one study.[135][136] There are numerous examples of patients that have been helped with physical therapy in the setting of acute neck

135 *Vincent et al. Systematic review of manual therapies for nonspecific neck pain. Joint Bone Spine 2013;80:508-15.*

136 *B. Hidalgo et al. The efficacy of MT and exercise for treating neck pain: A systematic review. Journal of Back and Musculoskeletal Rehabilitation 30(2017) 1149-1169.*

pain. The most straightforward answer as to why there is improvement is that acute neck pain resolves without treatment to some degree, and in most patients. It is hard to then separate the effect of physical therapy from the regular course of events (physicians call, the natural history).

However, beyond that, physical therapy appears to be effective when reviewing various clinical studies comparing neck pain improving both with and without physical therapy.[137]

One Theory For How Physical Therapy Works

There is no clear explanation for how physical therapy works. Generally, the favored theory is that increased joint movement due to stretching and exercise is thought to decrease muscle spasms in the affected joint. Then, due to negative feedback, pain signalling is decreased as there is more joint movement and less muscle spasms. This may seem very nonspecific (because it is), which attests to the difficulty in providing processes like this in a living organism.[138]

Can Physical Therapy Help Avoid Surgery?

The answer is yes. Strength-training, targetted physical training, and core muscle conditioning have been shown in numerous

---

137 *In a systematic review of research studies studies, manual therapy (including PT with manual therapy, which includes the goal of improving range of motion, and overlaps with spinal manipulation) manual therapy was shown to improve neck pain, and that combinations of manual/physical therapy and exercise were better than either treatment alone alone.*

138 *Bialosky JE et al. The mechanisms of manual therapy in the treatment of musculoskeletal pain: A comprehensive model. Man Ther. 2009;14:531-538.*

studies to effectively help patients avoid more expensive and invasive neck pain treatments, including surgery. Physical therapy complications are relatively few.

What Does Physical Therapy Consist Of?

Broadly speaking, physical therapy for neck pain includes three general categories of therapy in addition to numerous adjunctive treatments.

- *Stretching:* Helps maintain normal range of motion, provide relief for muscles in spasm due to abnormal posture, and muscle spasms from painful nerve irritation.

- *Dynamic Stabilization Exercises:* Dynamic stabilization entails exercises that rely heavily upon stabilizing muscle through various ranges of motion. One example of this would be using exercise balls, which require stabilizing core muscles to keep you balanced on the exercise ball.

- *Core Strengthening Exercises:* Traditional exercises that increase muscle bulk through the abdominal muscle group and posterior spinal muscles. One example of core-strengthening would be weighted-machine crunches and hyperextensions.

Key Points

- Prior to beginning a new exercise program, always discuss your plans with a healthcare professional.

- There are numerous physical therapy exercises, and further detail is beyond the scope of this book. The author recommends at the very least, a consultation with a physical therapist to obtain a professional evaluation and to develop a training program with goals in mind. This will help avoid injury maximize your chances of successfully completing your planned therapy.

- Keep this in mind: patients that complete a physical therapy program are less likely to seek out more invasive low back pain treatments.

- Having chronic back problems should not be regarded as a reason to avoid physical therapy. If you are concerned with injuring yourself during physical therpay, then a physical therapist can guide you safely through the process.

- Some chronic medical conditions, obesity/morbid obesity, and a lack of physical conditioning makes physical therapy challenging for some people. Physical therapists and their teams strive to help patients with these hurdles.

41 What Are The Different Kinds of Neck Injections ?

There are many different kinds of neck injections. This is an important topic that needs further explanation. At a certain point in the nonsurgical work-up, neck injections may eventually be considered as part of the treatment plan, depending on symptom severity and the persistence of symptoms despite physical therapy and other exercises. Other clinical factors may alter the recommendations and some will be discussed below.

Many patients are reluctant to undergo cervical injections. These are prudent individuals and if a cautious person visualizes this process, most reasonable people would be reluctant. However, to consider spinal surgery only and not injections is usually an opportunity for further education, as the chances of surgical success can be often be improved with injections, as well as the chances of avoiding surgery. Also, while cervical spine surgery is well-tolerated, the extent of potential complications and their severity of cervical spine surgery are much greater than that of an injection. The potential major complications of epidural injections can be freely downloaded in a literature review by Epstein.[139]

Upon learning that a patient has had a previous injection, the provider will always ask what kind of injection did they have, what level of the spine was the injection intended for, and the extent of any pain relief. Without providing this information, it is very difficult to confirm whether or not an injection will results in similar success or failure. Ideally, obtaining and bringing copies of procedural records are the best way to help avoid repeated injections that were unhelpful, and helps create forward momentum through the diagnosis and treatment process— Otherwise, every new consultant must reconstruct the entire history.

There is no method for a physician to truly know what kind of injection that one had, and the details provided by the patient are helpful in avoiding repeated studies, some of which may not have been historically helpful. Another myth is the statement that, 'injections didn't help before.' This generalization does not take into consideration the many forms of 'injections', or 'interventions' as they are called. And when patients consider saying that they did not have any improvement with injections and are not interested in any more, it must be determined what intervention was received. It is analagous to saying that medications were tried before, and no new ones will be tried, without having a list of which ones were

---

139 *Epstein NE. Major risks and complications of cervical epidural steroid injections: An updated review. Surg Neurol Int. 9:86, 2018.*

tried. Clinical histories are important.

In the subsequent section, the types of injections will be explained, and their benefits. It will become apparent in that section why they are useful in select instances, for both the diagnosis and treatment of pain for spinal conditions. Again, it is very helpful for the patient to know his or her entire treatment history in detail, including dates. Occasionally, patients will be asked for copies of their records. Likely said, it is hard to tell what type of an injection that one had if they are coming from an unfamiliar region and it is not well-known with types of injections are commonly offered, or pain management physician clinical patterns.

Anecdotally, motivated patients are more likely to get better. In the relatively less motivated patient a providers request to obtain records from a prior practice can seem like an unnecessary hurdle.[140] Furthermore, patients that cannot recall the names and locations of the practices they went to, or whether or not the injections were performed either months or years ago, are relatively less likely to improve. For patients with difficulty remembering these details, it is important to keep a log of what was said and done, with the date. The more information, the more helpful. There are patients with dozens of imaging studies, exhausted non-surgical treatments and other studies where after 10 years this information becomes quite complex. Therefore, keep a record of your care. Patients with notebooks tend to be more informed and do better. They write down questions and have more questions answered at a very opportune, short office visit. In the author's experience, one patient had a list of 40 questions written out.

Another reason why it is important to have a system for keeping track of your medical history and treatment history is to increase the chances of informed consent. Informed consent means that a patient understand the risks and benefits of a treatment, the risks and benefits of no treatment, and the entire process is understand

---

140 *Navratilova E and Porreca F. Reward and motivation in pain and pain relief. Nat Neurosci. 17(10):1304-1312.*

in detail in laman's terms to the fulleset extent possible, given the limitations of the situation.[141] Since the types of injections differ and the risks and benefits, if you want to project to a doctor that you fully understand the things that they recommend for you, one way to do that would be to demonstrate that you understood what was done to you in the past. And you do not have to remember everything, but having a process for writing these things down means that you do not have to memorize anything. And when you have questions for yourself and for other healthcare providers, you have written them down and you are able to look at your information. This also prevents you from having repeat treatments unnecessarily.

General types of injections for Neck Pain

Paraspinal Intramuscular
Epidural steroids - intralaminar
Epidural steroids trans-foraminal
Cervical facet
Rhizotomy

141 *Since the author's definition and scope of informed consent is fairly narrow, please see the American Medical Association's definition, developed by their legal team, and a full page long. After reading that, a more greater understanding of informed consent becomes possible. https://www.ama-assn.org/delivering-care/ethics/informed-consent*

Paraspinal muscle injections

The paraspinal muscle injection is by far the most common injection that patients have had, prior to an appointment with a spinal surgeon. Even if one does not have their records with them at the time of their appointment with the spine surgeon, statistically this is the most common injection obtained. This is because it can be performed without image-guidance (x-rays) making it common in a primary care office, neurologist office, or urgent care and emergency department setting.

There are two reasons why this injection is performed so often in the acute setting. First, it was mentioned earlier that paraspinal muscle strain is the most common cause of acute neck and low back pain. In the absence of any of the red flag symptoms that prompt a physician to obtain early advanced imaging, neck pain that does not radiate down to the shoulders and arms is most often due to muscle strain and therefore would relief with an injection of the muscles. Cortisol is one of many kinds of steroids that is injected into the muscle. The second reason why the injection is performed is that he requires very little advanced training and equipment because the muscles are just beneath the skin and complications are exceedingly rare. These side effects are limited to a local skin reaction to a component of the steroids, pain from steroid injection, and rarely, there are people that are allergic to the injection. Since cortisol is a synthetic version of the natural steroid that is in the body, it is more often that an additive is the cause of the rare allergic reaction that some people experience in assoication with the medication. This reaction includes hives, breathing difficulty, facial and facial swelling, and rarely, life-threatening respiratory problems. Moreover, sometimes the allergic reaction is due to the local anesthetic that is sometimes included with the steroid injection.

What are some of the advantages of steroid injections? Well the alternative form of steroids can be intravenous or oral, both of which are absorbed in far greater quantities throughout your body and long-term use of which can cause high blood pressure, weight gain, insulin resistance (pre-diabetes) and increased blood glucose('increased sugars'), decreased bone density (osteoporosis) and more.

Epidural Steroid Injection

An epidural steroid injections (ESI) decrease nerve inflammation in a more precise manner by allowing a concentrated delivery of steroids to the area adjacent to the inflammed nerve. The steroids that are used are synthetic versions of the steroids found in your body, that reduces inflammation. This can provide long acting relief for low back or neck pain, especially with associated arm or leg pain. Inflammation of the nerves is a common cause of this sharp, intense, neck and back pain radiating down the arm (radicular pain), often followed by a painful tingling sensation.

This procedure is performed in an office setting under minimal sedation and local anesthesia (the skin is temporarily made numb with an injection). This procedure is performed awake. Additionally, medication to alleviate pain and anxiety can be given during the procedure, in order to facilitate the study. Normally, this procedure is brief, and there is only some minimal bleeding, contained with a bandaid and some pressure, associated with the needle site. Often, the procedure provides dramatic pain relief and is long lasting.[142] This procedure is helpful in allowing many to avoid spinal surgery. Epidural steroid injections are considered to be the most effective non-surgical treatment of LBP or leg pain.

---

142 *Hassan KZ and Sherman AI. Epidural Steroids. StatPearls; published Jul 20 2020 in https://pubmed.ncbi.nlm.nih.gov/30726005/*

Epidural Steroid Injection- Transforaminal and Intralaminar njections

There are 2 approaches to a posterior epidural steroid injection: The intralaminar and transforaminal approach (Fig. 41-1). Typically, there are 2 reasons to perform one approach versus other. The first is the location of the source of nerve compression. For broad and central stenosis and nerve compression, and anterior/intralaminar approach is utilized. For foraminal stenosis, which is where the nerve root exits the spine, or in the region of the lateral recess, which is just prior to exiting the nerve root, a transforaminal approach is often preferred. However, in cases of severe neuroforaminal stenosis, some physicians may feel more comfortable with an interlaminar approach. A transforaminal approach in the cervical spine is more technically challenging and interlaminar injections are more universally practiced. Overall, there is no superior approach of the two, and there certainly is reserach that shows that there was no sginificant treatment difference.[143]

---

143 *Yoon JY et al. Cervical interlaminar epidural steroid injection for unilateral cervical radiculopathy: comparison of midline and parmedian approaches for efficacy. Korean J Radiol. 16(3):604-12. 2015.*

Selective Nerve Root Block

A selective nerve root block is more of a diagnostic procedures then a pain treatment procedure. The physician injects an anesthetic in combination with a steroid (for example, lidocaine), which temporarily blocks nerve transmission, shutting off pain and all other sensory transmission, including motor function in the muscle groups supplied by a particular nerve. Is this procedure safe? It has long been a concern that the selective cervical nerve root block was unsafe. Ma and colleagues in a large series of over 1000 patients that underwent these selective nerve root blocks found an incidence of minor complication to be 1.66%, which was only 14 patients. There were no catastrophic complications which could include damage to major vessels such as the neighboring vertebral artery that supplies blood to the brainstem, paralysis due to needle injury of the spinal cord, or death. In a randomized, double blind, controlled clinical study Riew and colleagues evaluated the effectiveness of selective cervical nerve root blocks finding that the use of the selective cervical nerve root block did not lead to a decrease number of patients needing surgery further cervical radicular pain.

Epidural Steroid Injections

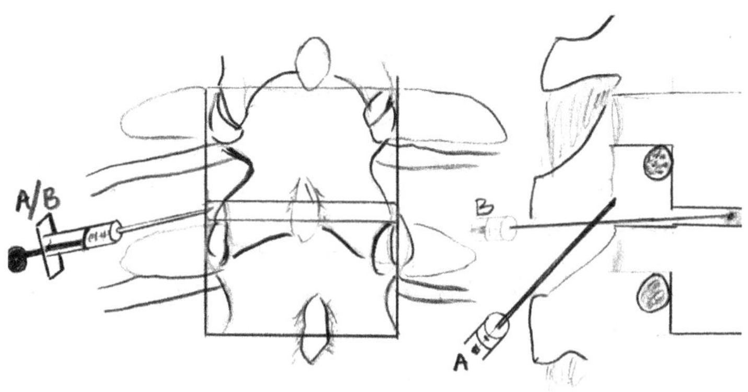

Figure 41-1. Cervical epidural steroid injections (posterior perspective of the spine, left, lateral perspective right). Diagrams simplified. Steroids can be delivered epidurally via the nerve foramen (left diagram, transforaminally), or intralaminarly, which is technically more straightforward (right diagram, A). Injections into the disc can also be safely approached (Path B in both diagrams above) for a variety of diagnostic and treatment tests, but is a less common therapy. The needle approach is guided by fluoroscopy (x-rays) and all nervous system tissue is avoided by the needle. These procedures are tolerated very well.

42 What Are Some Types of Cervical Epidural Steroid Injections?

A cervical epidural steroid injection guides steroids precisely to the area surrounding the nerve and epidural space (area around the spinal canal with the nerves and spinal cord) at the region of the neural foramen or posterior to the central canal (See previous figure).

For each procedure, x-rays are used to guide the needle to localize the appropriate level and also to avoid needle injury to the nerve root, spinal cord, and other vital structures. After using x-ray to confirm that the needle has reached the appropriate location, contrast dye is injected to confirm that the needle is outside of the dura. Contrast blocks x-rays from passing through it, the pain management doctor can confirm that the needle is in the appropriate space around the nerves, and then steroids and other medication can be delivered precisely where they are needed (Fig. 42-1). As mentioned in the imaging section, x-rays are an ionizing radiation, and through its exposure is a risk for developing cancer— Although the total exposure is minimal, it is still a cumulative cancer risk, adding up through your lifetime. The concept of cumulative cancer risk is illustrated by the numerous reserach studies of pilots and airline cabin crew- repeated exposures throughout time can lead to an elevated frequency of developing cancer.[144] Perhaps a more relevent subject of cumulative risk of cancer comes from long term observational studies of women diagnosed in adolescence with scoliosis, who, through the nature of repeated imaging throughout life, have a 5 fold increase in breast cancer, and adolescent scoliosis most frequently results in a thoracic region scoliosis, placing the breast tissue in the line of radiation for the periodic imaging.[145]

Some facilities use a CT scanner to provide very precise injections, but the amount of radiation exposure is significantly greater. The benefits of a more sophisticated imaging system over a fluoroscopic image has not been demonstrated in studies. Epidural steroid injections are helpful for pain caused by disc herniations and foraminal stenosis. Some studies show that patients can improve up to 6 weeks after an ESI and as will be shown, can help patients avoid surgery.

---

144 *Di Trolio R et al. Cosmic radiation and cancer: is there a link? Future Oncol. 11(7):1123-35.*

145 *Luan F et al. Cancer and mortality risks of patients with scoliosis from radiation exposure: a systematic review and meta-analysis. aug 27, 2020. PMID 32852591*

Cervical Epidural Steroid Injections

Inflammation of the nerve roots causes neck pain and pain shooting down the extremity (cervical radicular pain). An epidural steroid injection (ESI) is a pain procedure where medications are delivered near the point of nerve compression or inflammation via injection of steroids and sometimes other analgesic medications. This needle is guided by x-ray. Steroids when delivered in this manner, provide long acting pain relief for either neck or extremity pain, and typically have less systemic side effects when corticosteroids are taken orally. Delivery of the steroids, as in an ESI, is a short procedure performed in an office or ambulatory setting under minimal sedation. You will be awake for this procedure, but with medication to help limit discomfort. The pain relief from an ESI can help patients avoid surgery. A review of 26 randomized controlled trials found moderate evidence that patients that underwent ESIs were less likely to require surgery for *low back pain.*[146] While there is less evidence for cervical injections, there is good evidence that cervical ESI can help patients put off surgery. In a prospective review study of 98 patients with cervical radiculopathy who underwent cervical ESI, 80% were reported decreased pain and were able to avoid surgery at the 2 year follow-up.[147] Epidural steroid injections are considered to be the most effective non-surgical treatment of LBP or leg pain.

---

146 *Bicket MC, et al. Epidural injections in prevention of surgery for spinal pain: systematic review and meta-analysis of randomized controlled trials. Spine J 15(2): 348-62, 2015.*

147 *Lee S et al. Clinical outcomes of cervical radiculopathy following epidural steroid injections: a prospective study with follow-up for more than 2 years. Spine. 37(12):1041-7, 2012.*

Transforaminal Epidural Steroid Injections

There is relatively less evidence regarding the effectiveness of cervical ESIs when compared to the lumbar spine. However, Cervical intralaminar ESI (Fig. 41-1) are effective at reducing neck and arm pain symptoms for acute and chronic radicular pain. Transforaminal injections (TFESI) approach the spine from an oblique angle to the neuroforamen (previous figure, left diagram). Typically, the TFESI approach is loss commonly utilized in practice due to some potentially life-threatening complications related to arterial puncture which includes ischemic and hemorrhagic strokes in the spinal cord, brainstem, midbrain, pons, and cerebellum.[148]

The vertebral artery is very close to the target in the TFESI, which in part supplies all of those aforementioned regions of the central nervous system. Puncture of the vertebral artery and death during a TFESI has been reported.[149] To Improve safety of these procedures, CT-guidance[150] and the use of ultrasound[151] with fluoroscopy have both been reported to aid in confirmation of anatomy during the procedure.

While these reported complications are troubling, to say the least, many pain management experts prefer this approach in experienced hands because anatomically there is greater logic

---

148 *Tiso RL et al. Adverse central nervous system sequelae after selective transforaminal block: the role of corticosteroids. Spine J 4:468-74: 2004.*

149 *Rozin et al. Death during transforaminal epidural steroid nerve root block (C7) due to perforation of the left vertebral artery. J spinal Cord Med 24:351-55: 2003.*

150 *Wolter T. et al CT-guided selective nerve root block with a dorsal approach. Am J Neuroradiol. 31(10):1831-6, 2010.*

151 *Narouze SN et al. Ultrasound-guided cervical selective nerve root block: a fluoroscopy-controlled feasibility study. Reg Anesth Pain med. 34(4):343-8, 2009.*

that the that the targetted nerve will be treated, providing useful diagnostic information in addiotion to the therapeutic value.

In one study of 64 patients, 70% of patients were able to avoid surgery.[152] Although less studied, one possible advantage is the that the symptomatic nerve in question can be more precisely targeted, as the nerve exits in the foramina, which theoretically delivers steroids in a more precise manner. At this time, there is no clear evidence in favor of one technique over the other..

Selective Nerve Root Block

A cervical selective nerve root block (CSNRB) is a growing technique, used predominantly in acute pain reduction to delivered steroids in the TFESI route describe above in more than thirty thousand patients each year[153]. This technique is also described as a diagnostic procedure, where local anesthetics are combined with steroids, which temporarily blocks nerve transmission, to a regional, but also with the result of causing numbness and weakness until the regional anesthetic wears off. After the local anesthetic

---

152 *Costandi SJ et al. Cervical Transforaminal Epidural Steroid Injections: Diagnostic and Therapeutic Value. Reg Anesth Pain Med. 40(6): 674-80. Reeg Anesth Pain Med.*

153 *Wolter T et al. CT-Guided Cervical Selective Nerve Root Block With a Dorsal Approach. Am J Neuroradiol 31:1831-36. 2010.*

wears off, the steroids are not short-acting, and will continue to provide lasting relief for a period of several months. This can be helpful because if the regional anesthetic blocks the pain sensation entirely , this is felt to serve as evidence that the targetted nerve root is the pain generator.

Cervical Epidural Steroid Injection Procedure

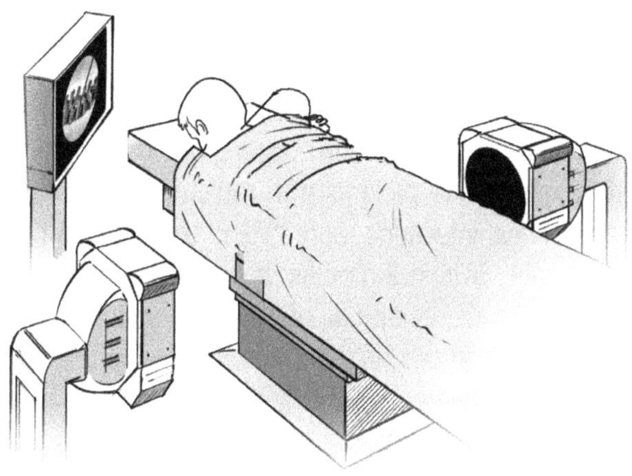

Figure 42-1. Illustration of procedure room layout. The patient is undergoing spinal injection (physician performing procedure removed from illustration). Using the x-ray machine in various orientations, the needle trajectory in relation to the spine can be observed on the monitor at the head of the patient's procedure bed. The patient is laying face down. There is a cutout for the patient to see through the bed. (adapted from Low Back Pain Guide, Weatherly Press 2019).

The Efficacy of Additional Spinal Epidural Steroid Injections

In the *Low Back Pain Guide*, for the lumbar spine, it was quoted that less than 10% of patients may benefit from repeat injections. However, there exists more promising reports that a repeat injection may be very helpful in obtaining pain relief for both a cervical and lumbar epidural steroid injection. Joswig and co-investigators evaluated 102 consecutive patients with radicular symptoms. Of those, 45 had cervical injections, and 85% of the patients had an improvement in pain. Within 2 months, a repeat cervical injection was performed on 6 patients and all of those patients had a satisfactory pain reduction. In fact, in the entire series, the pain reduction was signficant at one year, and only one patient with low back pain underwent a microdiscectomy.[154] Discuss this in advance with your surgeon, as the percentages are based on specific clinical scenarios, patients populations, definitions of success, and for very specific follow-up time points. These variables are carefully considered by your physician before deciding the risk - benefit ratio and offering a repeat procedure.

---

154 *Joswig H et al. Repeat epidural steroid injections for radicular pain due to lumbar or cervical disc herniation: what happens after 'salvage teratment'? Bone Joint J. 100-B*10):1364-1371, 2018.*

43 What is a Cervical Facet Injection?

Each spinal level[155] has a pair of posterior facet joints located on the right and left sides of the spine, which attach (via pedicles) to the anterior joint, the intervertebral disc. The facets aid in spinal stabilization and flexibility. The range of motion is dictated by the shape of the joint, and this shape is slightly different at each level. Degeneration and excessive loading of these joints is a result of (at least) our lifestyles, aging, and genetics. Facet joint degeneration may be evident at multiple levels, and it is not specifically evident on imaging which level may be contributing to the neck pain. For-

---

155 *The craniocervical or craniovertebral junction segments have unique anatomy which imparts a greater range of motion as well as greater degrees of freedom, and is the subject of books in itself. See Lopez AJ et al. Anatomy and biomechanics of the craniovertebral junction. Neurosurg Focus 38(4):E2, 2015.*

tunately, there is useful diagnostic and treatment method for facet joint pain.

This procedure is divided into two parts: a diagnostic injection, and in patients that have treatment relief, the nerve ablation, discussed in the next section. This procedure was first implemented in the lumbar spine, as axial low back pain without leg pain was far more common. This procedure has been is ideal for patients with similar features of facet joint pain. Predominantly axial neck pain, worse with extension of the neck, and usually without arm pain symptoms. Arm pain symptoms warrants further history and workup, but in the context of the spine, warrants a careful evaluation with MRI and other diagnostic tools.

Typical imaging findings include those of spondylosis. Often this is described as either 'hypertrophic facets', 'facet arthropathy', or less commonly 'facet degeneration.' A branch of the exiting nerve root, absent of motor or cutaneous sensation(skin sensation) exits and courses medially towards the facet joint, providing central nervous system feedback of the joint. These joints are relatively safer spinal structure to access from the posterior needle approach (Fig. 43-1). Local anesthetic is injected sequentially and the patient can provide feedback regarding the extent of pain relief.

Cervical Facet Joint Injection

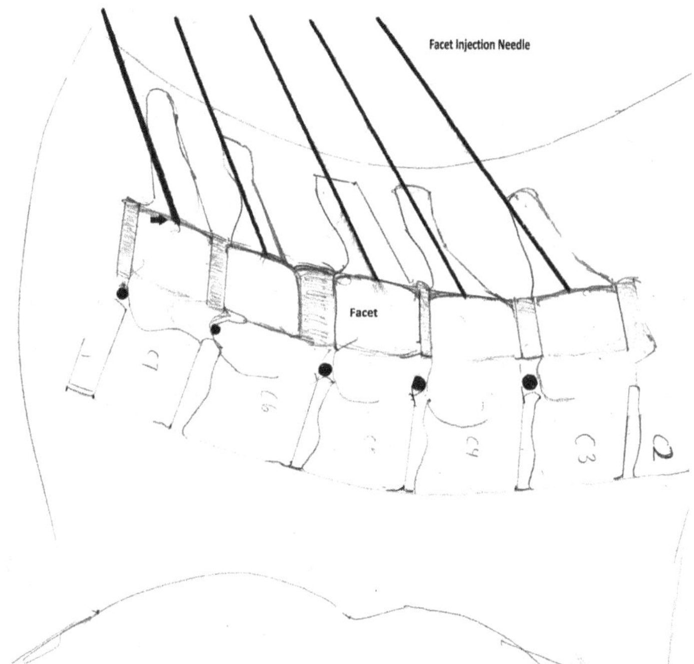

Figure 43-1. The Cervical Facet Joint Injection is a relatively safe diagnostic procedure that involves the injection of medial branch nerve bundles with local anesthetic. The patient can then determine how much pain relief they achieve before they choose to undergo ablation (destruction) of the medial nerve branches. Radiofrequency ablation of facet joints in the carefully selected patient provides excellent long term neck pain reduction in carefully selected patients.

44 What is Radiofrequency Ablation Helpful For?

In patients that have predominantly facet joint pain diagnosed by facet joint nerve blocks, radiofrequency ablation (RFA) is a very effective treatment.[156] Facet joint pain is predominantly pain confined to the neck, made worsened by any neck movement, particularly with extension of the neck, which places increased force on the facet joints. Less often, some extremity symptoms can be associated. With involvement of the upper cervical spine, associated headaches have been described. Typically, the diagnostic process for these headaches, referred to as 'cervicogenic headaches', is a prolonged process that can be expedited by a referral to a neurolo-

---

156 *Manchikanti L et al. Cervical zygapophysial (facet) joint pain: effectiveness of interventional management strategies. Postgrad Med 128(1):54-68, 2016.*

gist, to simultaneously explore additional causes of headache while concurrently undergoing workup for neck pain.[157] Radiofrequency ablation is another procedure involving needle placement in the posterior neck, but with up to several needles placed into the posterior facet joints. Due to the placement of multiple needles, and relatively greater chance of discomfort, some regional anesthesia is given (Fig. 44-1). In a review of 4 randomized trials and 6 observational studies a systematic review showed a benefit in favor of the use of RFA, but the quality of the evidence limited the strength of the recommendations to 'fair'. That is unfortunately a limitation that is commonly seen in neurosurgery and spinal surgery. However, a benefit is shown, whereas the indications for cervical fusion for neck pain are very nebulous. Many surgeons will not perform a multilevel anterior or posterior cervical fusion for neck pain, both due to the lack of literature support and the risk of life-threatening major complications. Again, an RFA should be attempted in the instance of chronic axial neck pain, failing all other conservative therapies, and without any other potential causes suspected on imaging. In another retrospective study, 64% of patients that underwent RFA were neck pain free at follow-up.[158] These are impressive results when one consider endpoints in most studies, which are usually not 'pain free' but rather pain reduction is the outcome measure. Success is often defined as a 'significant' improvement, and more recently a clinically significant improvement.[159]

---

157 *Shimohata et al. The Clinical Features, Risk Factors, and Surgical Teratment of Cervicogenic Headache in Patients with Cervical SPine Disorders Requiring Surgery. Headache. 57(7):1109-1117, 2017.*

158 *Duff P. et al Percutaneous radiofrequency rhizotomy for cervical zygapophyseal joint mediated neck pain: A retrospective review of outcomes in forty-four cases. J Back Musculoskelet Rehabil. 2991):1-5, 2016.*

159 *Today, whenever the word 'success' is used, it is helpful to know what the definition of success is. The definition used may not match your expectations. Also, the term 'significant' is nuanced in research. Significant can often be interpreted that a 'statistical' analysis was used in the study*

Of the interventional pain procedures, this one is relatively the most invasive, and still, this is a same day procedure. The only caveat is that some will perform the procedures in an ambulatory surgery center or hospital setting, still on an outpatient basis. The procedure begins with a local anesthetic to block pain fibers from different joints in the back. If a significant portion of pain is reduced then the medial branch nerves are ablated using radiofrequency generated by the tip of the instrument placed on the facet joints (other terms used in place of ablated are burned or lesioned). This is an excellent treatment for both neck and low back pain.

---

and it was determined that the difference (between two groups, e.g two treatment options, or treatment vs. no treatment) wasn't obtained by chance. However, there is considerable variance in statistical methods. One trend is for researchers to make a determination if a 'minimal clinical differnence' (MCD) was found between two groups. The MCD is usually a reference to a particular scale being used, e.g. a pain scale. The MCD is the number of paoints in the scale needed for a pain reduction to make a clinical impact for the patient. Prior research is usually done to determine this measurement. In other words, if a scale is out of 20, and the MCD is 3, then a reduction in 2 is most often not noticeable to the patient.

The following example should illustrate the value of the MCD. For one hypothetical study, the effectiveness of a neck pain treatment is being analyzed in a study, and the outcome of pain reduction is measured on a scale of 1-20, comparing patients with treatment to without treatment. The authors of the study conclude that significant pain reduction was achieved, which was that patients undergoing treatment had a score of 2.3 less. However, if the MCD is 3, then the difference isn't clinically significant (despite being statistically significant).

Radiofrequency Ablation

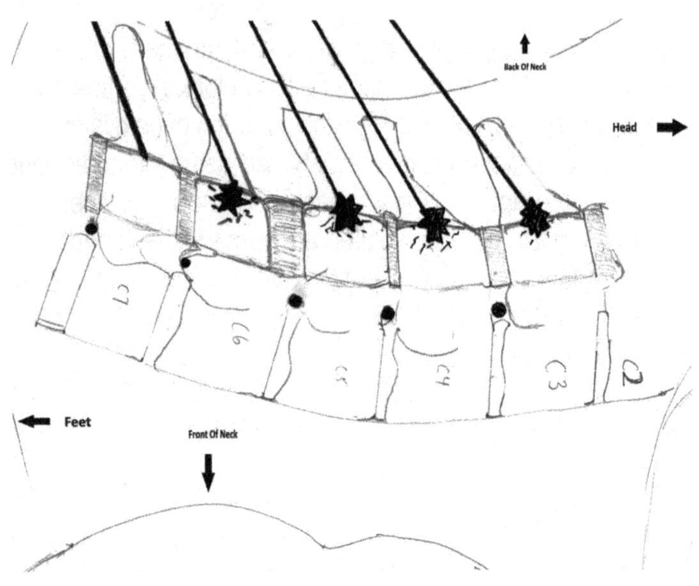

Figure 44-1. Radiofrequency ablation is a technique of neck pain treatment used by pain management physicians to lesion (destroy) nerve fibers to the facet joints. These fibers are previously identified in a separation procedure to be drivers of neck pain; during a cervical spinal facet joint block. This treatment of ablation is also commonly referred to as a rhizotomy.

SECTION V

SURGICAL TREATMENT

45 How Do I Know if I Need Surgery?

The short answer is that one will be unable to know for sure without a consultation from a spinal surgeon, and the advice of a primary care provider. The practice of medicine requires years of education and training to develop these skills required to answer questions like these. The more one can learn about spinal conditions and their respective treatment options, the better off they will be, because a more informed decision can be made.

In the persuit of becoming more informed through the internet, it is now very common to be exposed to personal reviews for just about anything offered in healthcare. These reviews are helpful as they educate us as patients to ask the best possible questions and to better understand a surgical procedure. However, a surgeon will not be able to explain why someone had a particularly good or bad experience, or why another patient had one type of surgery or not. Risk varies from patient to patient, and in order to maintain strict healthcare confidentiality, patient information will not be shared, ever.

Aside from that, while your risk of a complication varies depending on the type of operation you have, their are so many variables that come into play, it is beyond the scope of this discussion. Your surgical risk (complications), can be grouped into things that raise your risk (your medical, surgical, and social history), the planned operation (complexity of the surgery), and the postoperative period. A discussion with your surgeon should include a discussion of risk, as it will help you understand the nature of the surgery better.

Key Points

- Most people will not need surgery.
- Most people that require surgery for a degenerative condition of the spine should attempt to exhaust all nonsurgical measures before considering surgery.
- The right surgeon for a patient is someone they trust, have thoroughly had their condition and procedure explained to them, and appropriate expectations are discussed.

46 What Are the Roles of A Spine Surgeon?

The traditional role of a spinal surgeon has always been as a surgical consultant, who sees patients who were referred after a careful consideration that the spinal problem requires surgery as the principle means to getting better. A spinal surgeon has expertise in treating disorders of the spine surgically after careful consideration of appropriate nonsurgical management. In the majority of situations with early onset low back pain and leg pain, surgical intervention is not warranted. Therefore, a spinal surgery evaluation is not required up front.

With that said, the role has shifted over time for many spinal surgeons. Some surgeons provide many nonsurgical treatments and therefore are comfortable seeing patients without having had prior nonsurgical therapies such as physical therapy and epidural steroid injections.

The Comprehensive Care Clinic

Many 'comprehensive' care clinics use this distinguishing descriptor in the name of their business to advertise that all foreseeable treatments can be provided at one location. Overlooking the obvious appeal to business owners, this practice is also done in an effort to maintain continuity of care, apply a consistent philosophy of care across all spinal healthcare providers[160], limit pain by reducing wait times, and limit inefficiency through repeated studies. Many private and hospital-owned clinics aim to provide all services this way. With that said, the spinal surgeon in some instances is tasked to perform an evaluation of a patient and to make a determination what pathway of care the patient should then proceed. The general pathway involves making the determination if further diagnostic workup is required for the neck and back pain patient, and the goal is to make this as expedient as possible, while simultaneously working towards reducing pain. Next, after diagnosis, the decision is made as to which route the patient will take: nonsurgical or surgical pathway? This is just one of many business models. In order to maximize the public health benefit of their respective specialties, many surgeons are only able to see patients that meet all of the requirements for surgery. Finding this is out is just a matter of asking the clinic prior to your appointment.

---

160 *One example of a philosophy of care would be the common goal to limit opiate prescribing, to aid patients reduce risk factors for chronic spinal pain such as lose weight and quit tobacco products, and the use of nonsurgical treatment measures to the fullest extent possible.*

47 What is Minimally-Invasive Spine Surgery?

Minimally invasive spine surgery (MISS) is a general surgical principle describing the sparing soft tissue that must normally be mobilized from surgical corridor from the skin to the spine. The most popular method for this in the spine is used by using sequential dilators that dilates muscle. Until more recently, spinal surgery has had the reputation of being a painful type of surgery, with a long and painful recovery, due to the nature of the approach through muscle to reach the spine. Also, this degree of pain depends on a number of factors such as the patient's body weight and the distance from the skin incision to the spine, the purpose of the surgery (diagnosis), and the number of levels being operated on. and whether there was prior spinal surgery (extensive surgery in previously operated spinal levels typically causes greater postoperative pain). The traditional approach to the spine('midline approach') has typically involved a vertical incision in the middle of the back, where the muscles and soft tissues are split, and removed from the surface of the bone, where the muscles insert.

With the traditional approach, prolonged retraction under pressure is often required for the surgeon to have adequate view of the nerves and anatomy of the spine. At the end of the surgery, the muscle tension is released, but some of the muscle tissue will necrose (muscle cells will die, and atrophy) causing prolonged postoperative pain (Fig. 47-1). The muscular attachments cannot be reattached to the bone, and in many cases, most of the bone where the muscles attached do not have any bone to reattach to, because they were removed to accomplish the operation. With traditional surgery, this creates an area where fluid can accumulate, and increases the risk of spinal infection.

Minimally-invasive approaches use dilators to make an opening in the muscle where a tube the diameter of approximately two cm is used to approach the spine (Fig. 47-2). Small corridors are drilled through the posterior bony lamina and facet joint with very minimal removal of soft tissue and muscle, except from the point of insertion (Fig. 47-3). Large retractors that cause prolonged muscle pain are not used with MISS. As a result of dilating the muscle, the muscle falls back into position when the tube is removed, and there is no cavity where fluid collects(no drain is needed), lowering the risk of infection (Fig. 47-3).

Surgeons debate the exact definition, and some medical societies have defined MISS. If fusion surgery is planned for you, minimally-invasive surgery might be helpful for you. In select patients, minimally-invasive alternatives are becoming available for many procedures. Often minimally-invasive surgery may not be an option for you and at the time of this writing, there are not MISS alternatives for every surgical problem.

Posterior Cervical Midline Surgical Approach

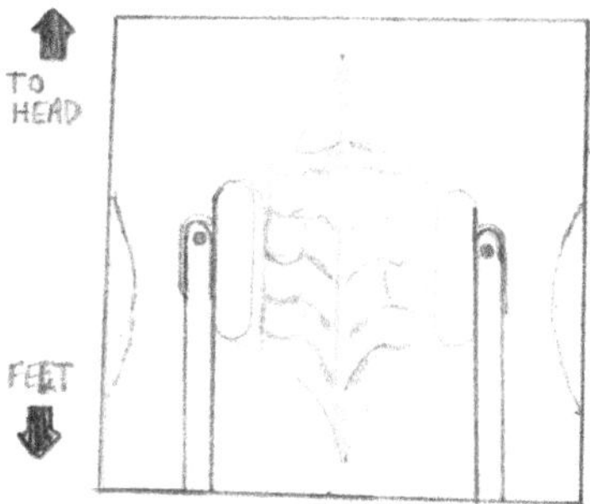

Figure 47-1. Traditional Midline Posterior Cervical Exposure involves a larger, midline incission and is typically suitable for multilevel cervical surgery. Exposure of the majority of the posterior cervical spine can be seen in this figure with a midline incision along the posterior neck.

Posterior Cervical Minimally-Invasive Approach

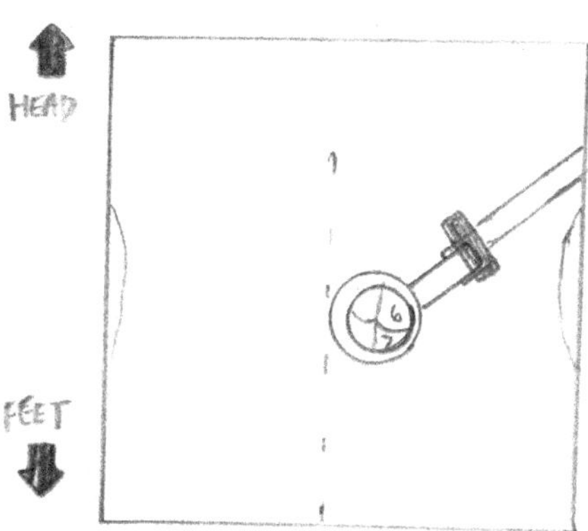

Figure 47-2. Minimally invasive surgery involves dilators that expand the muscle, rather than removing them from the point where they insert into the bone. For the most part, this results in less postoperative pain, and less wound healing complications. Since less of the spine is seen during surgery, x-rays are taken in the operating room to visualize the spine.

Tubular Approach, Expanded View

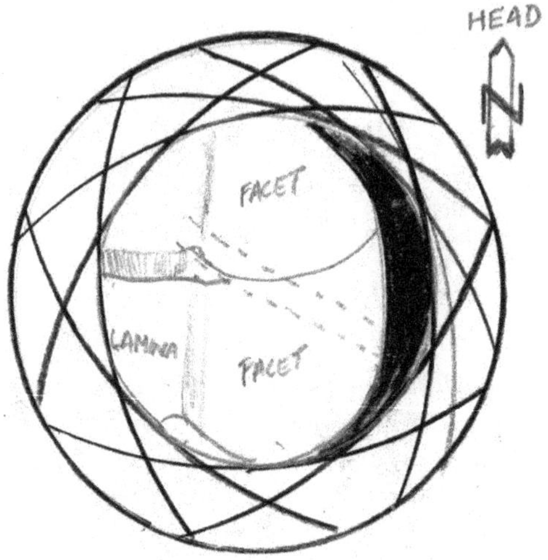

Figure 47-3. The tubular approach view is shown under magnification. A portion of the right-sided facet joints of two levels are seen as they meet the junction of the right-sided lamina, which covers the spinal canal. With training, this anatomy makes sense to the surgeon in allowing for a decompression of the nerve root that is just beneath the bone. Great care is taken not to injure the nerve or spinal cord, or destabilize the spine by the removal of significant portions of the facet joints.

Posterior Cervical Minimally-Invasive Approach With Tubular Retractors

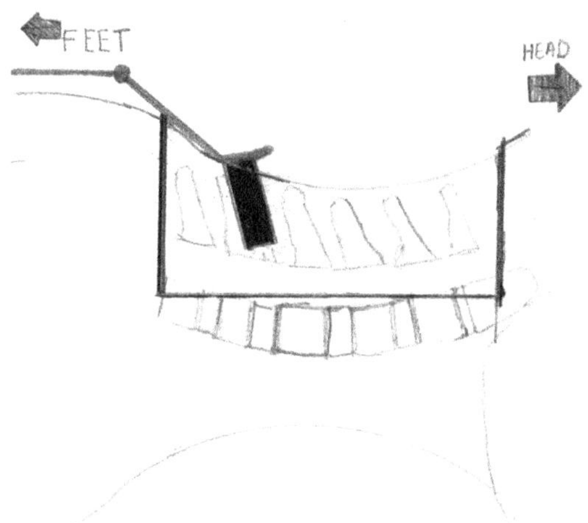

Figure 47-3. The posterior cervical spine is accessed through a tubular retractor as in the above figure. In this diagram above, the patient is facing down, with arrows indicating orientation of head and feet. As seen in this side view of the neck, the dilator spreads the muscle and soft tissue, without permanently disrupting the muscular attachment ot the bone. This 'subperiosteal' disruption results in decreased blood flow to the surgical site and the risk of wound healing complications and surgical site infection. At the end of surgery, the tube is removed, and the tissue collapse in place, obliterating the channel that was created to the spine. This is an advantage over the midline approach to the spine, where the cavity for spinal exposure is not obliterated.

48 What is Cervical Laser Spine Surgery?

Laser spine surgery refers to the placement of a laser in the center of a disc, which in turn creates heat that burns the center of a disc, and results in shrinking the disc, and facilitates the disintegration and evacuation of disc material both via aspiration and the use of an rongeur via and endoscopic port (Fig. 48-1). The ultimate goal is to relieve nerve root compression. The endoscope channel is the narrowest channel among the surgical procedures.

Another term for this procedure is the thermonucleoplasty. In the mid- to late 1990's, success in small clinical case series was reported using the Nd:YAG and Ho:YAG laser systems. This resection of the nucleus pulposus also lends to the procedure to be referred to as a nucleoplasty, which is essentially the same procedure, which, by definition, is also an endoscopic discectomy (Fig. 48-1). Overall, the quality of literature is limited to retrospective studies, which are not ideal for making generalizations of effectiveness. However, successful outcomes are generally reported.[161]

Mechanism of Nerve Decompression In Cervical Laser Spine Surgery

Cervical laser spine surgery includes several steps, and so there are a few ways that nerve roots are relieved of compression-by direct and indirect means. Entry to the disc space is thought to immediately decrease the intradiscal pressure and relieve nerve root compression. Next, central disc material is removed, which further decompresses the nerve by indirect means. When the anatomy facilitates direct decompression, the nerve and disc fragment are safely viewed, and the disc can be resected through the endoscopic working channel. Stenosic can also be decompressed via a foraminotomy. This is a direct decompression component. The decreased disc pressures result in the overall decrease in the pressure of the disc. Increased intradiscal pressures from disc collapse is a driver of symptomatic nerve compression and neck and arm pain. Descreased intradiscal pressure can be accomplished through a channel created by a needle through the annulus and into the center of the disc space. The medical literature is replete with short term perioperative success via clinical case reports. However, a summary of the medical studies has shown mixed results.

Due to the technical demands of this procedure, generally limited experience in the literature, and increased risk of perioperative complications, cervical endoscopic spinal surgery is limited to a very select few spinal surgeons.

---

161 *Epstein N. Percutaneous cervical laser diskectomy, thermoannuloplasty, and thermonucleoplasty; comparable results without surgery. Surg Neurol Int. 8:128, 2017.*

Posterior Endoscopic Cervical Foraminotomy and Discectomy Approach

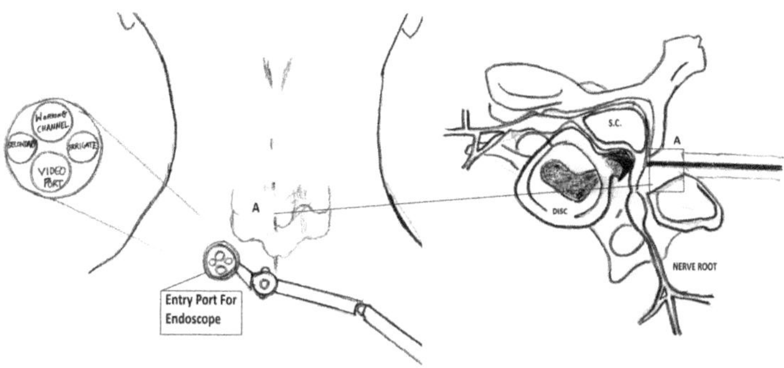

Figure 48-1. The posterior endoscopic cervical approach to the disc entails a posterolateral skin incision on the side of the herniated disc. A retractor arm holds the endoscopic working tube in place to prevent migration of the dilator tube. This is the penultimate minimally invasive approach, with some working channels advertising a 5 mm skin incision. The cervical foraminotomy is carried out with a high speed drill in the usual manner to access the herniated disc and disc space. At this point, when laser spine surgery is advertised from a posterior approach, a probe is inserted into the center of the disc to disintegrate and aspirate the nuclear material, and decrease the disc pressure and nerve compression.

49 What is a Discectomy?

A discectomy entails the removal of disc material. In the cervical spine, in practice, this typically is performed by an anterior cervical discectomy and fusion. In an anterior cervical discectomy, the entire disc is removed to reach the herniated posterior portion that is compressing the nerve (Fig. 49-1). This destabilizes the cervical level and an anterior cervical discectomy is followed by a structural graft or cage placement, which restores the normal lordotic cervical curvature, and keeps pressure off of the exiting cervical nerves on both sides of the spine. After the cage is placed, a plate spans the disc space, along with screws which affix (Fig. 49-2) the plate to the vertebral body above and below to eliminate motion, and allow for fusion to occur, which is slower biologic process whereby bone grows across the disc space to create a permanent bridge (Fig. 49-3).

An anterior cervical discectomy begins with an incision on the front of the neck, usually in a crease, to make the incision as cosmetic as possible. There is limited soft tissue and the spine can be easily exposed. Due to the lack of significant muscle disruption, The anterior cervical approach, (along with MIS posterior) approach have relatively less postoperative pain. This is very commonly an outpatient surgery.

Anterior Cervical Discectomy Approach

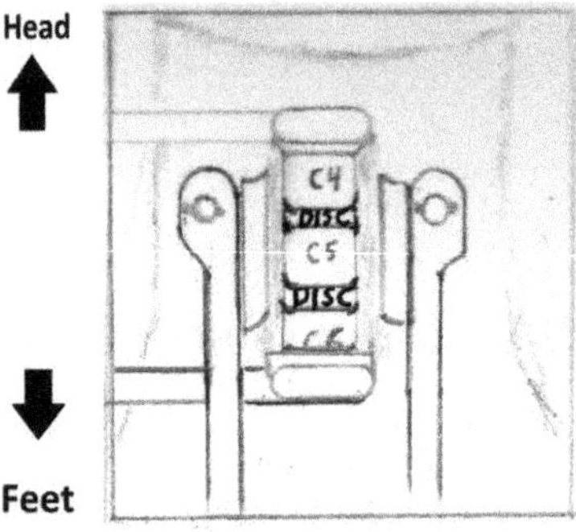

Figure 49-1. The anterior cervical approach is common, well-tolerated surgical procedure performed generally performed as an outpatient procedure (for 1 and 2 level cervical discectomy and fusions).

Common Postoperative Issues With The Anterior Approach

A detailed discussion of every complication imaginable is the subject of whole textbooks. In general, the retractors put pressure on the esophagus and trachea to expose the spine, and temporary swallowing discomfort and hoarseness are the most common complications encountered (See Figure Below). Major complications are rare. However, there are numerous major vascular, neurological, and visceral structures of which injury has been reported, and fortunately are very rare. The incidence mortality in one series was 1 out of 1015 patients, due to an esophageal injury.[162] While this is 'routine outpatient' surgery, these reports are still a reminder of the seriousness of surgery.

Smoking is an inhibitor of succesful fusion, which is the growth of bone across the graft and permanent elimination of motion at that level. Smoking has been shown to increase the risk of a multitude of postoperative complications, and in some regions, insurance companies will not authorize certain elective surgeries without lab testing proving that there is no nicotine in the blood prior to surgery.[163] Evidence suggests that it is not just the free radicals generated from smoking, but the nicotine as well. More detailed work is required. The association between nicotine exposure and pseudoarthrosis (impaired fusion) is more prominent in animal studies. While animal studies are helpful, they are not considered definitive evidence of a cause-effect relationship in people for a number of reasons.

Indeed, clinical studies are necessary, because often contradictory results are obtained when the same exposures are analyzed in human subjects. For further thought-provoking consideration, a number of common drug exposures in animal research studies, used perioperatively in routine spinal fusion procedures, have been shown to decrease fusion rates. Two notable exposures are vancomycin[164] and opiates.[165] Again,

---

162 *Fountas KN. Anterior cervical discectomy and fusion associated complications. Spine 32(21):2310-7, 2007.*

163 *Berman D et al. The Effect of Smoking on Spinal Fusion. Int J Spine Surg. 11(4):29, 2017.*

164 *Mendoza MC et al. The effect of vancomycin powder on bone healing in a rate spinal rhBMP-2 model. J Neurosurg Spine. 25(2):147-53, 2016.*

165 *Jain N et al. Opiods delay healing of spinal fusion: a rabbit posterolateral lumbar fusion model. Spine J 18(9):1659-1668, 2018.*

absolutely no conclusions can be made without well-designed clinical studies.

Anterior Cervical Fusion: Graft/Cage Placement Restores Original Disc Height Which Indirectly Decompresses Exiting Nerve Roots

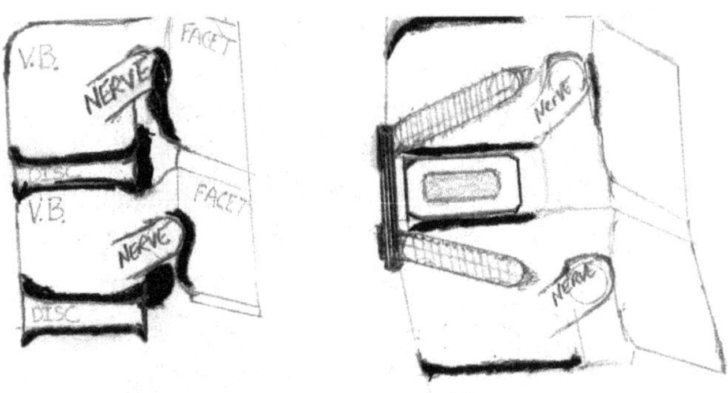

Figure 49-2. Anterior Cervical Fusion for persistent nerve compression due to spondylosis. Cervical foraminal stenosis (lateral view of the spine) results from a combination of facet and ligamenetous hypertrophy as well as posterior disc herniations (left image). After removal of the disc and osteophytes, A cage packed with bone is placed in the disc space to restore the cervical lordotic alignment (natural curvature). To keep the graft in place and to eliminate motion that would prevent fusion whereby bone grows across the graft from one endplate into the next, a plate is anchored to the two vertebral bodies (v.b.) with screws (right image). While the procedure is technically called a fusion, the actual fusion process takes months. Nicotine greatly impairs this process.

Fusion Is The Formation Of A Permanent Bridge of Bone Across A Motion Segment, and Takes Months

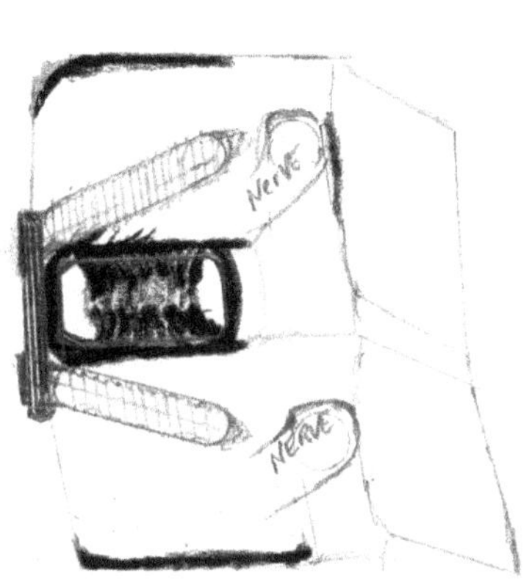

Figure 49-3. Anterior Cervical Fusion for persistent nerve compression due to spondylosis, 3 months after surgery, which demonstrates the growth of bone through the interbody cage. The cage is packed with bone and other substrates that enhance the success of fusion. Other factors that increase the chances of fusion include the absence of smoking, absence of osteoporosis, and excellent biomechanical fixation, securing the hardware and resistant to various forces such as flexion, extension, side bending, translation, and rotation.

50 What is a Posterior Cervical Decompression (Foraminotomy and Laminectomy Explained) ?

A laminotomy is a spinal procedure where part of the lamina is removed over the spinal canal in order to relieve symptoms of nerve compression. This can be performed in a number of ways. A foraminotomy can be combined when there is further nerve root compression. When there is enough encompression, a laminectomy is performed, which is the complete removal of the lamina. A hemilaminectomy is a complete removal of half of the lamina and a hemilaminotomy is in practice used interchangeably with a laminotomy, as they both refer to a subtotal portion of the lamina. A laminoforaminotomy refers to part of the lamina and facet to decompress the exiting nerve root. When specific requirements are met, after a laminoforaminotomy, a soft disc herniation can be removed, avoiding the need for an anterior cervical fusion (Fig. 50-1). There is no definite answer as to which is superior, an anterior cervical fusion or a posterior laminoforaminotomy with discectomy. In practice, the location of the compression must be compatible with the surgical choice. Decompression without fusion is the most common surgery to treat stenosis in the lumbar spine, but the safe access to the disc space is limited in the neck, and therefore, most surgeons prefer the anterior cervical fusion. Anecdotally, there are a few surgeons that perform alterative anterior approaches to perform nerve root decompressions. One in particular, called the 'Jho procedure', has been reported. It is one of the relatively rare procedures being practiced in spinal surgery, but if one is interested it would not be hard to learn more about the procedure and who may be offering this option. Very serious complications have been reported, but not in every publication. It is likely that there is a very steep learning curve for this procedure, meaning that the risk is very high in relatively less experienced hands (maintains a low complication rate after a certain number of procedures are performed). There are strong proponents that contend that the anterior cervical foraminotomy('Jho Procedure') is a safe procedure and in many ways has its advantages when directly compared to the posterior foraminotomy.[166] One such advantage is the theoretical argument that anterior foraminotomy is less likely to result in destabilization of the cervical spine, and require fusion later on. A posterior foraminotomy, is generally not recommended in patients with cervical a kyphotic alignment, as there is a significant risk for worsening kyphosis and neck pain. This stems from the removal of lamina and part

---

166 *Kim S et al. Comparison of Anterior Cervical Foraminotomy and Posterior Cervical Foraminotomy for Treating Single Level Unilateral Cervical Radiculopathy. Spine 44(19):1339-1347: 2019.*

of the facet joints, which are essential to the preservation of the alignment. In traditional open procedures, the removal of larger portions of bone has been observed even more often to result in post-laminectomy kyphosis, or subluxation and instability. This is rectified with the placement of screws and rods at the levels of bone removal (Fig. 50-2).

Minimally- Invasive Posterior Cervical Hemilaminectomy and Right-Sided Foraminotomy With Discectomy

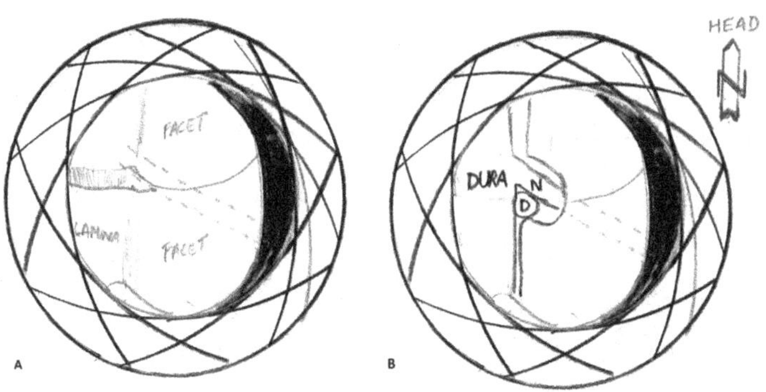

Figure 50-1. Minimally-invasive posterior exposure of the lamina and facet of two adjacent levels of the spine (A). The lamina has been drilled on one side to expose the underlying dura. A small portion of the facets joints have been resected to expose the exiting nerve root. A compressive soft disc herniation can now be removed with care, which is compressing the exiting nerve root (N). This location below the exiting nerve is referred to as the axilla of the nerve.

Stabilization And Fusion May Be Needed Depending On The Extent of Decompression

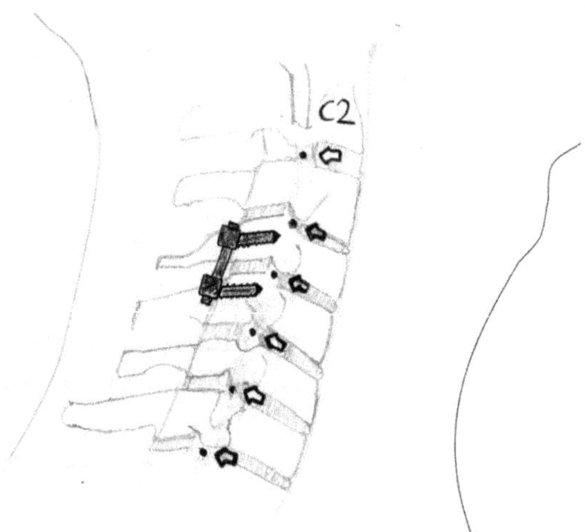

w

Figure 50-2. Depending on the severity of your nerve compression, not only is the lamina removed from the center of the spine, along with the underlying ligaments, but a significant amount of the facet from each side. Considering the amount of bone resected and the cervical alignment, the surgeon may decide that a posterior fusion is required. Seen above, screws are placed in the remaining facet joints of C4 and C5, which is called a lateral mass fusion. See the following section for more details about a fusion. The 2 screw are placed on both sides of the spine, for a total of 4 screws, with each pair connected by a rod. This serves to eliminate motion at C4 and C5 and allow for bone to grow across the joints of C4 and C5 (C4-C5) to provide permanent stabilization.

M

51 **What is a Spinal Fusion?**

Spinal fusion surgery is a surgical procedure where hardware is placed in the spine with the goal to facilitate the growth of bone across (fusing) a segment of the spine. The goal of a fusion is to remove motion entirely across a joint. This 'segment' that the bone grows across is a region where motion normally has occured (Fig 49-3).

There are several indications for fusion surgery. Often, in the lumbar spine, this can be used for spondylolisthesis, disc herniations that recur after a prior discectomy, scoliosis, and spondylolisthesis due to pars fractures (spondylolysis). There are many more indications for fusion surgery and these can be thought of as any situation where there is abnormal and painful motion in the spine, or where enough bone will be resected that abnormal and painful motion may occur after the procedure is performed. One good example of this is seen in scoliosis due to degenerative disc disease. In this type of scoliosis, the disc degenerates on one side first, causing uneven loading of your body weight onto the side of the disc collapse, resulting in degeneration of multiple discs, all on the same side, resulting in a a spinal curvature (scoliosis). The ligaments and facet joints respond to the stresses of this abnormal curvature causing growth of the joints and thickening of the ligaments, which in turn can compress nerves. As you can see, if you were to remove the joints and ligaments to relieve painful nerve compression, the pain might be relieved temporarily, but the spinal curvature will increase resulting in worse scoliosis and more severe nerve root compression. The treatment then is a decompression followed by a fusion.

Instrumentation and Fusion

Bone will best grow across a motion segment of the spine with a scaffold of bone that the surgeon places across the segment that is being fused. Surgeons often use donor bone (processed and treated bone from a cadaver) because there is inadequate bone from the spine to use for the fusion procedure.

Fusion and Nonfusion

The rates of fusion have improved over time with improvements in the hardware that provide more rigid fixation of the spine, and the guidance systems that allow for precision placement of the hardware. The fixation hardware will not withstand the stresses of the-body forever. It was quickly realized that bone is more likely to grow across an area of motion, if it is stabilized with implants that connect the area above and below the region of motion. If the bone does not fully grow across this area of motion, the daily stresses on these implants could lead to loosening of the implants, cage or screw migration with painful nerve compression, or rod and screw breakage.

How New Technology Might Impact Fusion

The evolution of implants has been a process of improving implant design to achieve the following desirable characteristics: increased durability, increased stability, and increased safety of placing the implants into the spine. Many factors affect the likelihood of bone fully bridging across an area of motion. Fusion can occur anytime within three to twelve months.

Often, bone removed to decompress the nerves is saved and used for the fusion mass. Also, this bone is frequently not enough, and donated bone (allograft) is also placed in the fusion site. There are many alternative products to facilitate the fusion, including proteins and cells that are thought to stimulate fusion and synthetic bone which is rich in calcium and minerals thought to support the fusion.

An in-depth discussion of fusion techniques and considerations such as implants and fusion supplements are well-beyond the scope of this book. However, understanding specific risk factors for not having a fusion(called pseudoarthrosis) such as tobacco use, is an important discussion to have with one's physician.

Key Points

- Fusion(arthrodesis) consists of two time frames: a surgical component and the process of fusion, where bone bridges across an immobilized region of the spine.
- In fusion surgery, a surgeon immobilizes a region of the spine with screws and rods, a plate, or some other implant that results in no movement across a previously mobile area. The screws and rods are typically are not removed.
- Over the next 3 -12 months, bone cells slowly grow across this fusion bridge and bone is deposited.
- While a fusion results in less range of motion, the overall goal is to maximize one's quality of life.

52 What Are Some of the Most Common Risks of Cervical Spine Surgery?

Every surgery has a risk of a complication. Since each patient has a unique medical and surgical history, this discussion is best left to a detailed discussion that you should have with your surgeon.

It is important for you to understand that the term risk and the term 'complication' can have a variable meaning. Instead, ask yourself what your expectations of surgery are, and see if the surgeon has the same expecations as you do. Then determine what are the things that can happen in surgery, and after surgery. Then, see if there is any long term risks. Long term risks from a fusion could involve a failure to fuse, possibly rod breakage, or symptomatic narrowing at the adjacent level of the spine, or even persistent pain without improvement.

General Complication Categories: Preoperative, Intraoperative, and Postoperative

One helpful way to group complications in your mind, and to assist you in asking the most helpful questions is to think of the complications that can occur. When it comes to degenerative disc diseases that require surgery, there are relatively less preoperative complications to consider. One way to help you conceptualize these general groups is to use the example of a patien that needs a lumbar discectomy, but uses a blood thinner to prevent blood clots. The patients doctor tells them that stopping coumadin carries the risk of forming other blood clots. So, a requirement of most spinal surgeries by most spinal surgeons is to stop blood thinners several days before surgery. This is to make the surgery safe and prevent major bleeding. The preoperative complication risks come from stopping the blood thinner. The likelihood of having this problem varies, depending on the reason for needing blood thinners. In surgery, abnormal bleeding may still occur, depending on the blood thinner. Major blood loss would be an intraoperative risk. Postoperatively, restarting the blood thinner is necessary due to the blood clot risk. There is no guidance as to exactly how soon it can safely be started after surgery. If it is started too soon, the risks are developing a large collection of blood in the wound itself(hematoma) and possibly severe pain or a neurological problem from compression of nerves by the hematoma. This would be an example of the postoperative risk. Not all examples of risk and complications occur before, during, and after surgery, like the example of blood thinner use. Howevere, this is a great example to illustrates how your unique medical issues impact your chances of having a complication, and this can occur at any time before, during, or after surgery.

General Examples of Surgical and Medical Risks of Spinal Surgery[167]

•Infection

•Persistent or worsening pain, or limited duration of pain relief

• A need for further spinal surgery

•Blood loss requiring a transfusion

•Pneumonia

•Blood clots (deep venous thrombosis, or DVT)

•Failure of fusion

•Accelerated degeneration at the normal disc below or above a fusion at the adjacent segment (called adjacent segment disease)

167 *This is a brief list and a consultation with a healthcare professional is required for a detailed discussion of the risks and benefits of any medical therapy. A recurring theme throughout this book is that many medical details that can influence one's likelihood of having a particular desired or undesired outcome.*

53 **Can a Cervical Disc Be Replaced?**

Cervical disc replacement can be interpreted as disc regeneration or be replacement with an artificial disc. Cervical disc replacement has been available as an FDA approved treatment for greater than 10 years, and there are a good number of surgeons trained in this technique. When a patient has chronic arm pain and concordant nerve root compression due to a disc herniation and/or compressive osteophytes and has failed nonsurgical therapies, surgical options from an anterior approach most commonly include anterior cervical fusion and cervical disc replacement. Anterior cervical fusions are an almost universal treatment and are well tolerated.

There is one major advantage to a total disc replacement, and that is the concern that there will be a loss of motion. Loss of range of motion is noticeable to the patient, and a significant difference has been observed as compared with before surgery and after plating.[168]

The advantages to this surgery, which is upheld by studies, is

---

168 *Lee JH et al. Comparison of cervical kinematics between patients iwth cervical artificial disc replacement and anterior cervical discectomy and fusion for cervical disc herniation. Spine J 14:1199-1204, 2014.*

that a cervical disc replacement is motion-sparing (Fig. 53-1). **The two treatments, anterior cervical fusion and anterior cervical disc replacement, are similar in terms of clinical effectiveness at up to 10 years when utilized in the manner prescribed during the FDA trial.** Another important question medical experts have been closely looking at is for any evidence that disc replacement slows down the rate of adjacent segment degeneration.

Adjacent Segment Degeneration: Fusion Versus Disc Replacement

After a cervical fusion, it has been observed that due to the rigid fixation of the disc space, the range of motion decreased at the level of the surgery (big surprise), but increased at the levels above and below.[169] This finding and other biomechanical data and subsequently numerous proscopective clinical studies have found the rate of adjacent segment degeneration requiring reoperation to be occuring at a relatively unchanged rate of 2.3% per year. This was even more likely in patients that had anterior and posterior combined surgeries, a similar finding in the lumbar spine, and likely thought to be due to the increased stiffness of the spine next to the mobile adjacent disc.[170] When analyzing data pooled together from two FDA device trials, as early as 7 years out from the initial surgery, patients that underwent cervical disc replacement had fewer second surgeries at the adjacent level.[171] However, over

---

169 *Eck JC et al. Biomechanical study on the effect of cervical spine fusion on adjacent-level intradiscal pressure and segmental motion. Spine. 27:2431-4, 2002.*

170 *Lee JC et al. Risk-factor analysis of adjacent-segment pathology requiring surgery following anterior, posterior, fusion, and nonfusion cervical sine operations: survivorship analysis of 1358 patients. J Bone Joint Surg Am. 965(21):1761-7, 2014.*

171 *Ghobrial GM et al. Symptomatic adjacent level disease requiring surgery: Analysis of 10-year results form a prospective, randomized, clinical trial comparing cervical disc arthroplasty to anterior cervical fusion. Neu-*

time, more data should come to light.

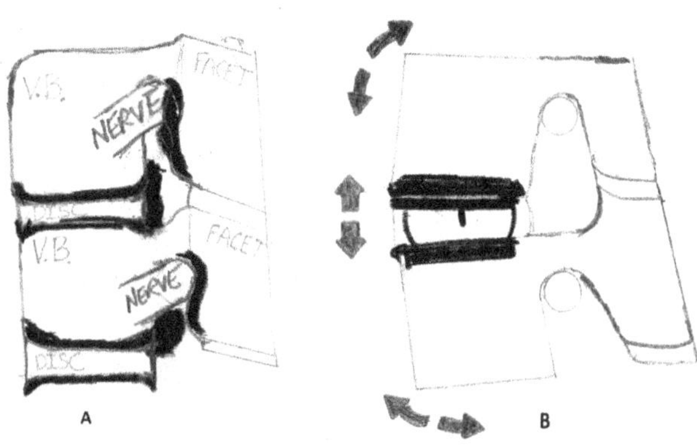

Figure 53-1. Anterior Cervical Disc Replacement, an alternative to anterior cervical fusion, is FDA approved for 1 or 2 level cervical spondylotic disease (A) with cervical radiculopathy after a trial of conservative management. The advantages of cervical disc replacement are preserved neck motion, and potentially the delay of the onset of symptomatic adjacent segment degeneration requiring surgery, a problem that occurs at a regular rate of approximately 2.3% per year.

---

rosurgery. 84(2):347-354, 2019.

54 Can Surgery Help Me If I Have One Isolated Cervical 'Disc Problem' (Found on MRI)?

From a statistical standpoint, it is not suprising that if someone were to obtain a cervical MRI in 2020 that they could conclude that he or she has a 'disc problem'. Yet, a disc herniation, disc bulge, disc extrusion, disc protrusion, degenerative disc, and/or disc sequestration are incredibly common and as discussed earlier in this book, it is so common that odds are, if a 40 year-old without symptoms were to get a cervical MRI, they are more likely than not to have one of these findings identified by the radiologist. This includes a diagnosis of degenerative disc disease. Therefore, it is difficult to conclude if this is a problem or not.

When pain is the only symptom, and the problem is thought to be a cervical disc herniation, it is best to attempt all available nonsurgical therapies that are within your means. Most disc herniations will improve on there own, and surgery is rarely required early-on in the first three months. There are exceptions such as neurologic deficits (see Ch. 8). Physical therapy is the most common initial recommendation for back and neck pain. However, most people do not have a budget that accomodates for an extra 80 dollars, several times a week. Numerous other nonsurgical therapies have arisen out of an understanding that not all treatments work best for every patient. However, when it comes to treatments for a isolated cervical 'disc problem'- which is usually referring to cervical degenerative disease with neck pain, and no arm pain symptom, surgery is the last resort, regardless of the patient.

First and foremost, it cannot be recommended at this time by the author. However, this is a controversial indication, meaning, there is still ongoing debate amongst surgeons, and that fusion for cervical degenerative disc disease, solely for neck pain symptoms (absence of attributable arm symptoms) may not result in improvement.[172] Historically, this has not worked in the past. The surgical success rate is low. Surgery carries risks, and no matter how rare a certain complication might be, it still occurs.

In summary, while research has not conclusively shown that surgery is a great option for isolated cervical disc disease, speak to your surgeon and discuss your options with him or her.

---

172 *Sugaware, Taku. Anterior Cervical Spine Surgery for Degenerative Disease: A Review. Neurol Med Chir. 55(7):540-546, 2015.*

55 Can Spinal Surgery Help Isolated Neck Pain ?

Neck pain is most often due to muscle and ligamentous strain and sprain. It is a very common problem. There are many conditions that are less common that can cause neck pain, but for the majority of people, neck pain is due to overuse injuries involving the muscles of the neck. Injuries to the ligaments are less common and require more force to injure. Spinal degenerative conditions play a major role as well. Arthritis in a joint, is most often a pain that is due to chronic motion, the 'wear-and-tear' condition. What kind of surgery would help neck pain in that case? It would be a motion stabilizing surgery. The reasons why many surgeons do not offer surery for isolated neck pain thought to be caused by a spinal degenerative conditions is several. For one, it is very debilitating. It entails a fusion operation where metal implants are used to hold the joints of the neck in fixed alignment. Because degenerative disc disease involves multiple levels, the surgery could require the use of implants- a fusion- which increases the risk of having a complication. These risks are significant. Pain caused by degenerative disc disease could be caused by inflammation arising from disc spaces and the neighboring tissues across multiple spinal levels. Examples of pain generators also include the cervical facet joints and cervical discs (discogenic pain), and/or painful muscular and ligamentous strain.

It is important to know that any structure in the neck, base of the skull, and compartments of your chest can cause neck pain. It is not possible to reliably come at a diagnosis just by characterizing your painful symptoms. Please review the section on red flag symptoms which are features of neck pain that should prompt you to seek an urgent evaluation by a physician.

56 Is Mobile Phone Use Associated With Neck Pain?

Reflecting on the past two decades, one of the many fascinating transformations that the world has witnessed has been the widespread adoption of cellular phones. According to a Pew Research Study, in the United States, cell phone ownership among adults has increased from 80 to 96% and smartphone use increased from 35 to 81%![173] Improvements in national cellular and broadband infrastructure have increased the relevance of mobile phones in our daily lives, with one 2019 study estimating that on average, U.S. adults spend nearly 4 hours each day on their smartphones, surpassing time spent on the television for the first time in 2019.[174]

---

173 *https://www.pewresearch.org/internet/fact-sheet/mobile/ results last updated June 12, 2019.*

174 *https://www.emarketer.com/content/average-us-time-spent-*

One driver of the increasing number of minutes spent each day using a mobile device has been attributed to improvements in text messaging, internet browsing, and the rapid adoption of social media use through mobile phone applications. As a consequence of this, concerns have been raised about the potential for an increase in the frequency of neck pain in the general population; a condition called 'text neck'. *Text neck* has been described as the neck posture necessary to read a phone that is at the level of your chest. It has been theorized that prolonged neck flexion accelerates wear and tear on the cervical spine. Most of us are familiar with the discomfort with prolonged durations of keeping the neck flexed while using a mobile phone or PDA. Surgeons are one group with an occupation that find themselves spending hours a day with the neck flexed. Some have acknowledged this activity as a high risk for developing neck pathology.

Neck flexion can range from 15 to 50 degrees, as observed during cell phone use.

Biomechanical studies have all yield both similar findings that increased neck flexion leads to increased stresses on the cervicothoracic spinal region. Torque increases the further down the cervical spine you go, as the neck is flexed. While this force cannot be measured in a person, it is estimated that the pressure on the neck can reach a maximum of 60 pounds at 60 degrees.[175]

Other observational studies show a correlation between cell phone use and neck and upper back pain. Gustafsson and colleagues followed 7000 young adults aged 20-24 for 5 years, finding a correlation with neck pain and mobile phone use.[176] To be fair, studies exist that have not found an association between text neck posture and neck pain. In 2018, conducted in Brazil, of 150 young adults

---

with-mobile-in-2019-has-increased, published June 4, 2019.

175 *Hansraj KK. Assessment of stresses in the cervical spine caused by posture and position of the head. Surg Technol Int. 25:277-9, 2014.*

176 *Gustafsson E et al. Texting on mobile phones and musculoskeletal disorders in young adults: A five-year cohort study. Appl Ergon. 58:208-214, 2017*

aged 18 to 21 found no association between neck posture, texting, and neck pain frequency. [177]

Text Neck – Biomechanical forces

Degrees Flexion	Force (in pounds)
15	27
30	40
60	60

Conclusions

Although medical evidence shows an association between cell phone use and neck pain, this if far from certain. It is very difficult to arrive at this conclusion as control subjects, which are people who do not use cell phones, are hard to come by these days. Also, neck pain is very common, reported long before cell phone use, and today as well. **At the present time, there is no definitive link between smartphone use and neck pain (text neck).** However, poor home and workplace ergonomics and other practices that require constant neck flexion are very often associated with patients seeking treatment for neck pain. This pain is often relieved by limiting chronic neck flexion, which as we have shown above, decreases rotational forces on the lower cervical spine.

177 *Damasceno GM et al. Text neck and neck pain in 18-21 year-old young adults. Eur Spine J. 27(6):1249-1254, 2018.*

57 Is There a Role for Stem Cell Injections To Treat Neck Pain, or Even Reverse Disc Degeneration?

At the time of this writing, there is no role for cellular injections into the cervical spine, or anywhere in the spine, for that matter. Cellular injections is a much more broader term than stem cells, and why that matters will be discussed below. The procedure to inject cells into the disc space is increasing in popularity in affluent markets outside of the US. Now, the use of cellular injections are creeping into the US market, with claims of being able to relieve neck or low back pain, and to halt or reverse disc degeneration (Fig. 57-1). This may come to as a surprise as it is becoming more common in other aspects of healthcare. The fact of the matter is, no clear role has been established for the administratiuon of any cellular therapy as of 2020, and therefore these drugs are manufactured outside of FDA oversight, potentially exposing yourself to serious health risks by circumventing expensive manufacturing standards. Not only that, while this technology is outside of FDA oversight, a growing body of evidence suggests that needle insertion into the disc space results in accelerated disc degeneration and decline in appropriate functioning.[178]

Cellular Therapy

Cellular therapy is a broad catch-all phrase referring to any cell, whether it be taken from your own tissue or harvested from a donor. The topic of stem cell injections creates even more confusion than the nature of degenerative disc disease. There are many reasons for this confusion. First, stem cells are generically advertised to patients. That is because the stem cell therapies are not FDA approved, and therefore not required to be more specific. In truth, what is being offered are cells, but not *stem* cells.

This distinction does matter, as a stem cell can develop into any cell and continue to divide without end. In the lab setting, with under the optimum conditions, the cells can replicate for an unlimited time.

Indeed, cancer cells replicate without end, and this unceasing replication is one of the deadly concerns of stem cells.[179] In the lab, stem cells are cultured and with the correct signals (chemical signalling), they are *differentiated* into precursors, which are intermediate cells that can then differentiate into one of several types of

---

178 *Korecki CL et al. Needle puncture injury affects intervertebral disc mechanics and biology in an organ culture model. SPine. 33(3):235-41, 2008.*

179 *Rando TA, Stem cells, ageing and the quest for immortality. Nature 441, 1080-1086:2006.*

mature cell types.

Obstacles to Providing Therapeutic Relief Via Intradiscal Cellular Therapy

There are numerous obstacles to providing a benefit with cell injections into the intervertebral disc. First and foremost, before discussing them, there is limited research to suggest this procedure works, and therefore it is experimental at the time of writing. The description of the process of disc degeneration should clarify the matter and illustrate the obstacles to cell regeneration via cell injection.

Intervertebral Disc Degeneration: A Cascade of Molecular, Biologic, and Structure Changes

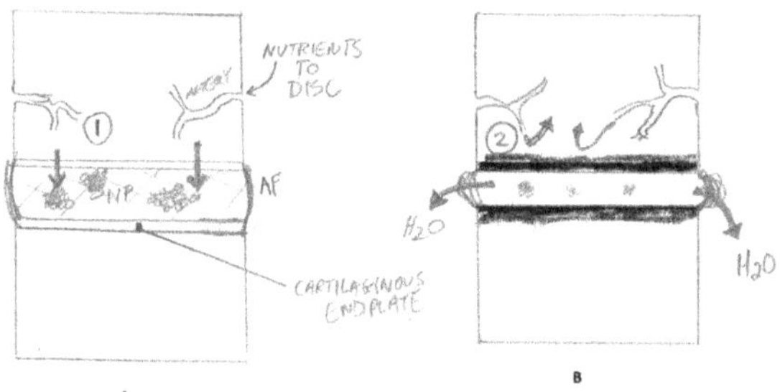

Figure 57-1. Intervertebral Disc Degeneration begins with water and proteoglycan loss in the nucleus pulposus, the center of the disc (labeled NP, on left figure). Nutrients are delivered to the cartilaginous endplate by segmental vessels and their branches (1). The nutrients then diffuse across the endplate to the NP, where chondrocytes (cartilaginous cells) generate the matrix of proteoglycans that bind water and contribute to the favorable

biomechanical properties of the disc space. The loss of water is ongoing, and this leads to a loss of disc height and biomechanical support, resulting in increased endplate inflammation and sclerotic changes (calcification), which in turn leads to decreased diffusion of nutritients to the chondrocytes). For a review of the detailed molecure, structural, and cell mediated chemical signaling changes, these reviews are abundant and available online.[180]

Cellular Injection Into the Disc Space

One problem with using cellular therapy to treat cervical disc degeneration is maintaining cell viability. As seen in the figure above, disc degeneration is seen with calcification of the endplates and decreased nutrient supply to the cells. This decreased nutritent supply is irreversible and there is no way to confirm cell viability.[181] Therefore, the cells are being injected into a degenerated cervical disc throught the standard approach, but without any clinical support that the cells will appropriately 'graft' (Fig. 57-2).

Ideally, the cells will be able to use the available nutrients, generate proteoglycans, and restore volume to the nucleus pulposus and restore disc height, and in turn, stabilize the disc level and decrease neck pain. However, clinical studies are required.

The next unanswered question is the ideal cell type that will lead to this reversal of degeneration. A form of partially differentiated or mature chondrocyte makes sense, and a stem cell can form just about any cell type in the body, and is a risk for cancer as well. injection into the degenerated disc musc cultured long enough, these cells become mature cells, which are hard to distinguish from

---

180 *Smith LJ et al. Advancing cell therapies for intervertebral disc regeneration from the lab to the clinic: Recommendations of the ORS spine section.*

181 *Erwin WM et al. The cellular and molecular biology of the intervertebral disc: A clinician's primer. J Can Chiropr Assoc. 58(3): 2014.*

the fully developed cells in your body, and many of which either do not divide or they have a limited number of times the cell can divide.

Lastly, for viable cells to be safely transferred into the disc space they have to come from a culture that is handled meticulously to prevent bacterial contamination. Discitis, or infection of the disc is a very serious risk that has been reported in patients receiving an intradiscal injection of any kind.[182] When procedures are not FDA approved, they are unlikely to have been manufactured in a setting that has met the stringent requirements set by the FDA. Aside from infection this means exposing yourself to unsafe chemical additives and stabilizers, that normally would not be an issue with an FDA approved product.

One of the many other numerous concerns arises regarding auto-immunity, which occurs when receiving a transplant. The disc space does not have a blood supply, and it receives nutrients via diffusion as described above. It is not well known how the disc will react to foreign cells. One way to overcome this would be to harvest tissue, then, in a lab setting, differentiate the tissue into the intermediate (progenitors) cell types, and then reinject them into the donor (called an autotransplant). Ultimately there is no good answer to this question.

182 *Subach BR et al. Epidural abscess and cauda equina syndrome after percutaneous intradiscal therapy in degenerative lumbar disc disease. Spine J. 12(11)e1-4: 2012.*

Intradiscal Injection Of Cellular therapy To The Disc Space

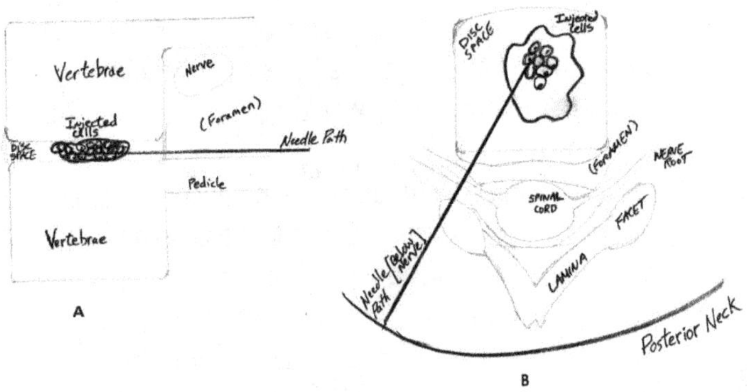

Figure 57-2. Intradiscal 'Stem Cell' Injections: Two views showing needle trajectory and delivery of cellular therapy to disc space. This treatment is experimental and not FDA approved at this time of this writing.

Conclusions

In summary, cervical disc degeneration is a complex process involving structural, biomechanical, and cellular changes. The theory of cellular regeneration is promising, but is unproven. One needs to be very cautious about the specific treatments that are being offered, as there are serious life-threatening risks with any spinal procedure. This is particularly the case with non-FDA approved treatments. Considerable research is underway and the author looks forward to a time when 'restorative' treatments are part of the spinal treatment armamentarium.

Selected Bibliography

- Back and Neck Pain, McCarberg, Stanos, D'Arcy (Oxford, 2012).
- Back Pain by Loren Fishman, M.D., and Carol Ardman (Norton, 1999).
- Chiropractic: The Superior Alternative. William Koch. (Bayeux Arts, 1995).
- Neck and Arm Pain, Rene Caillet, M.D. (F.A. Davis Co., 1964)
- Neck and Back Pain. Christopher Jenner (How To Books, Ltd, 2011).
- Neck Pain: Medical Diagnosis and Comprehensive Manage ment. Borenstein, Wiesel, and Boden (W.B. Sauders Co., 1996).
- No More Neck Pain! 9 Step Program for Your Neck, Shoulders and Head. Heike Hofler (Sterling, 1999).
- The End of Back Pain by Patrick A. Roth, M.D.
- The Neck Pain Handbook: Your Guide to Understanding and Treating Neck Pain. Grant Cooper, M.D. and Alex Visco, M.D. (DiaMedica, 2009).

- What To Do For A Pain In The Neck by Jerome Schofferman, M.D. (Fireside, 2001).

Selected Internet Resources

- www.spine.org/knowyourback: This is a great spinal education resource and is provided by the North American Spine Society, which is a large multidisciplinary medical organization focusing on education, research, and both evidence and value-based spinal care.

- www.spineuniverse.com: A great tool for patients and health-care providers regarding the lastest treatment options, as well as education about the spine, common spinal problems, and all of the surgical and non-surgical treatment options.

- https://smiss.org/patient-resources: For patients that want to learn about the latest cutting edge, and minimally-invasive surgeries, run by an educational society. Excellent educational information on cervical laminoforaminotomy, endoscopic discfectomy, minimally-invasive (MIS) lateral approach, MIS lumbar microdiscectomy, MIS tubuluar microdiscectomy, MIS TLIF, percutaneous pedicle screw instrumentation, and pre-sacral approach.

- https://radiopaedia.org/ Is an 'open-edit' educational reference created by radiologists and other related health professionals with the goals to promote education. They have the largest free library of case imaging, which is well organized, as well as educational articles. While this is one of the most useful websites for spinal imaging education, the material is most often targetted towards physicans. However, it is free to use and can undoubtedly improve one's understanding of the field, regardless of some of the drawbacks.

- https://www.ncbi.nlm.nih.gov/books This website of the National Center For Biotechnology Information (NCBI) provides free review 'e-books' on numerous clinical subjects. This material is accessible to anyone. No account is needed and can be downloaded as a PDF file. This is updated and reviewed material and contains content that is equivalent to very expensive textbook chapters.

- https://www.fda.gov/medical-devices The US Food and Drug Administration regulates the use of spinal implants and medications in the United States. Detailed information regarding approved indications, reports, recalls, and other notices can be freely located here.

Selected References

1.Bressler HB, Keyes WJ, Rochon PA, Badley E. The prevalence of low back pain in the elderly. A systematic review of the literature. *Spine (Phila Pa 1976).* 1999;24(17):1813-1819.

2.Pengel LH, Herbert RD, Maher CG, Refshauge KM. Acute low back pain: systematic review of its prognosis. *BMJ.* 2003;327(7410):323.

3.Docking RE, Fleming J, Brayne C, et al. Epidemiology of back pain in older adults: prevalence and risk factors for back pain onset. *Rheumatology (Oxford).* 2011;50(9):1645-1653.

4.Demyttenaere K, Bruffaerts R, Lee S, et al. Mental disorders among persons with chronic back or neck pain: results from the World Mental Health Surveys. *Pain.* 2007;129(3):332-342.

5.Qaseem A, Wilt TJ, McLean RM, Forciea MA, Clinical Guidelines Committee of the American College of P. Noninvasive Treatments for Acute, Subacute, and Chronic Low Back Pain: A Clinical Practice Guideline From the American College of Physicians. *Ann Intern Med.* 2017;166(7):514-530.

6.Summaries for patients. Physiotherapist-directed exercise, advice, or both for low back pain. *Ann Intern Med.* 2007;146(11):I56.

7.Hagen EM, Odelien KH, Lie SA, Eriksen HR. Adding a physical exercise programme to brief intervention for low back pain patients did not increase return to work. *Scand J Public Health.* 2010;38(7):731-738.

8.Machado LA, Maher CG, Herbert RD, Clare H, McAuley JH. The effectiveness of the McKenzie method in addition to first-line care for acute low back pain: a randomized controlled trial. *BMC Med.* 2010;8:10.

9.Rubinstein SM, Terwee CB, Assendelft WJ, de Boer MR, van Tulder MW. Spinal manipulative therapy for acute low-back pain.

Cochrane Database Syst Rev. 2012(9):CD008880.

10.Rubinstein SM, Terwee CB, Assendelft WJ, de Boer MR, van Tulder MW. Spinal manipulative therapy for acute low back pain: an update of the cochrane review. *Spine (Phila Pa 1976).* 2013;38(3):E158-177.

11.Konczalik W, Elsayed S, Boszczyk B. Experience of a fellowship in spinal surgery: a quantitative analysis. *Eur Spine J.* 2014;23 Suppl 1:S40-54.

12.Grabel ZJ, Hart RA, Clark AP, et al. Adult Spinal Deformity Knowledge in Orthopedic Spine Surgeons: Impact of Fellowship Training, Experience, and Practice Characteristics. *Spine Deform.* 2018;6(1):60-66.

13.Clark AJ, Garcia RM, Keefe MK, et al. Results of the AANS membership survey of adult spinal deformity knowledge: impact of training, practice experience, and assessment of potential areas for improved education: Clinical article. *J Neurosurg Spine.* 2014;21(4):640-647.

14.Pejrona M, Ristori G, Villafane JH, Pregliasco FE, Berjano P. Does specialty matter? A survey on 176 Italian neurosurgeons and orthopedic spine surgeons confirms similar competency for common spinal conditions and supports multidisciplinary teams in comprehensive and complex spinal care. *Spine J.* 2017.

15.Boden SD. The use of radiographic imaging studies in the evaluation of patients who have degenerative disorders of the lumbar spine. *J Bone Joint Surg Am.* 1996;78(1):114-124.

16.Boden SD, McCowin PR, Davis DO, Dina TS, Mark AS, Wiesel S. Abnormal magnetic-resonance scans of the cervical spine in asymptomatic subjects. A prospective investigation. *J Bone Joint Surg Am.* 1990;72(8):1178-1184.

Acknowledgements

I would like to thank my wife Michelle and my three boys for their love and support. I also would like to thank my father for his guidance and encouragement. I would like to thank my colleagues for their support. Neurosurgery is a small medical community and I am indebted to my colleagues who have shared their insight and valuable perspectives on modern spinal surgery treatments, which I have incorporated into this manuscript.

A

B

C

D

E

F

H

I

K

L

M

O

P

R

S

T

X

www.ingramcontent.com/pod-product-compliance
Lightning Source LLC
Chambersburg PA
CBHW031422270326
41930CB00007B/542

* 9 7 8 1 9 4 9 1 4 8 0 3 9 *